Text written by Marta M. Mobley, on behalf of Story Terrace and Mary Farrell
Design Grade Design & Adeline Media
Copyright © Mary Farrell

www.marymcmillan.com

First print April 2020

StoryTerrace

www.StoryTerrace.com

~Mary McMillan~

The Mother of Physical Therapy

WRITTEN BY
MARY FARRELL AND MARTA M. MOBLEY
ON BEHALF OF MARY MCMILLAN

CONTENTS

CONTENTS *cont.*

AUTHOR'S NOTE

This biography is written from Mary McMillan's many letters home to her family, as well as her diaries and writings during her work and world travels. In addition, the authors used the journals she wrote during the time she was held captive in two Japanese Internment camps. Also included are her personal photos and memorabilia from her life, work, teaching, and leadership of Physical Therapy during the period of 1919-1959.

PART ONE
1885-1915

1

"I LEARN TO SUCCOR THE UNFORTUNATE"

The reader might wonder what drove me to dedicate my life to helping people who were suffering and to become known as "The Mother of Physical Therapy." My family might say it was due to the illness and sudden loss of my loved ones at an early age. The colleagues I worked with for over 40 years wrote it was in my nature to step right in to ease a patient's misery and offer my sincere dedication, hard work, and vitality to our great profession. My hundreds of dear Physical Therapy students would have shared that I inspired and nurtured within them to offer their best healing abilities to their patients—but I believe it was the Almighty who placed the fire inside me that blazed my destiny—which led me on my multifarious journey from my birthplace of Boston, to Liverpool, back to America, then onto China, Manila, Shanghai, and finally back home again. What I want to confess most to those who read my story, is that I knew from an early age I was meant to heal and assist those who suffered and were in pain, and that I was fearless and unafraid to help as many of them as I could, no matter the peril.

I was born Mary Jeannie Livingston McMillan the fifth child of my full-blooded Scottish parents when my father Archibald McMillan turned 40 years old and my mother Catherine McMillan Livingston was 39 years old. My three brothers—Archibald, born on January 10, 1871 in Dumfriesshire, Scotland; John William, born March 2, 1875; Edward Neil, born on July 12, 1877—were all born in Boston, Massachusetts and Lillie A. was born August 12, 1879. Baby Lillie died on January 1, 1880 at only five months, 21 days old.

They considered me a miracle baby on November 28, 1880 because I was born so closely after the death of my sister, Lillie, only eleven months after her tragic death. Imagine the wonder and surprise to my brothers when their feisty, bright, brown-eyed baby girl sister had the spirit of a Scottish warrior.

Much of the person I became had been fused together by a combination of my family lineage, early childhood tragedy and varied cultural experiences. This trifecta greatly influenced the important work I pursued in my life.

My family immigrated to America from Scotland in 1873. They moved to Hyde Park about eight miles southwest of Boston. We lived at 21 Charles Street where my father set up a tailor shop, Archibald and Sons, located 101 Tremont Street in Boston. My brothers apprenticed with our father in the family shop.

Our Scottish ancestors had been immigrating to America since the 1600s when men and women who adhered to the Protestant faith were welcomed to the thirteen New England Colonies besides South Carolina and Virginia. The only way to immigrate to the United States was to sign a contract to become an indentured servant. Some Scots also came over because of their defeat with the English in the Battle of Culloden in 1746. Then came the Financial Panic in Europe in 1873 and the level of unemployment soared. The United States gave my parents the ability to immigrate as assisted immigrants, my father as a skilled worker via their family members in Canada.

Our family grew from the deep roots in the lands of the Scottish Highlands. My father was born in Argyll, Scotland, whose Gaelic people are distinguished by their clan's colors and tartans. This area is one of the most Celtic counties in the Highlands and was ruled

12

by Ian Campbell of Islay in the 1800s, a man of noble character and the greatest landowner clinging to the romantic traditions of our country.

When one sees Scotland in their minds, visions of cliff sided clusters of small islands offering verdant green hillsides and mountains, rock quarries, crags and free-flowing streams that savagely curve their way through the moorlands. The area was harsh with cold lands to tame, but with the strength, stubbornness, and perseverance of our Scottish ancestors, we did just that.

The longstanding Gaelic oral tradition has passed on through our family history and ancient stories handed down from generation to generation. Our Scottish ancestors battled as painted warriors, unafraid to fight and lose their lives for their family, friends, and lands. Add that of the Vikings and Irish people's blood to the Scottish DNA, those rebels who invaded our lands created a fine mix of brave, courageous, hardworking, and stubborn Scots.

Each family clan who originated in the area, from the MacArthurs to MacNaughtons, to the MacDougall and MacCallums, to the MacGregors and MacDonalds, and to my family, the MacMillans, were great Scottish people. My father's ancestors raised their families in the Killean and Kilkenzie, which name derived from St. Killian and Irish Missionary Bishop and used for cattle, hogs, sheep, beans, peas, and oats traced back to the early 1700s.

The Killean and Kilkenzie parish where my father and his family were raised was on the northern boundary, near a stream where two vital churches were erected in 1787 and 1825, which served a population of 2,000 people in the area. Their people suffered much hardship, but persevered despite their difficulties.

The Sept of Clan MacMillan's motto is *Misesrissuccereredisco*, "I Learn to Succor the Unfortunate." The origin of our family name, MacMhaolain, meant "Son of the bald" or "tonsure done. " They descended from Airbertach, a Hebridean prince of the royal house of Moray.

The MacMillans and their descendants of Gilchrist "Maolan" settled in Kintyre throughout the Middle Ages, and the immediate descendants of Alexander of the Cross who on record were the royal tenants in the Mull of Kintyre in the early sixteenth century. Alexander WS of Dunmore (1698-1770) spent much of the wealth he accumulated in his legal practice buying up estates in Kintyre, upon which he settled many of his relatives and more distant clan connections.

The McMillians were at one time a clan of importance but became dependents to the Campbells when the crown gave their lands to their rival clan. The M'millans therefore gave their loyalty to MacMhaolain Mor a Chnap who remained loyal to the Lords of the Isles who fled Kilchamaigin South Knap. Following the loss of Knapdale many M'millans settled to the south in Kintyre, much of which remained M'donald territory for a century before also falling to the Campbells.

The Campbells and MacNeills oversaw Knapdale until the year 1775, when Sir Archibald Campbell Invernie purchased the estate. My father's family was part of the Campbell Clan family and named after the long lineage of Lord Archibald Campbell's in Argyll of Inveraray Castle.

My mother, Catherine Livingston, was born in Glasgow, Scotland, to her father, John Livingston, born in 1815 in Cragnish, and Mother Jeanie, called Jane McKenchnie, was born in Oban, a small resort town in Argyll and Bute. She had two sisters, Mary, two years younger, and Jane, six years her junior. I was named after her beloved sister, Mary. The children were raised in Glasgow in the St. George Parish in the county of Lanarkshire, one of ten parishes in the area at that time.

14

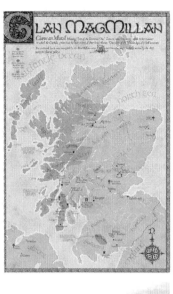

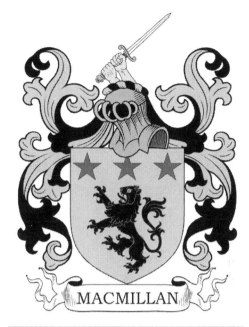

MACMILLAN

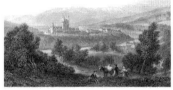

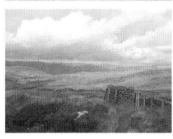

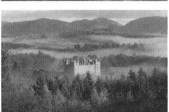

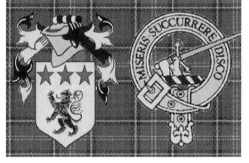

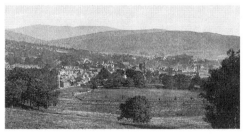

*Map of the Scottish Highlands, McMillan clan coat of arms
and motto, family tartan and scenic highlands*

February 16, 1884 was the day my childhood would change forever. I was four years old when I sensed the happiness in our home shifted into melancholy and sadness. I remember it being very cold when my mother went into labor with her sixth child. It was a very difficult birth, and she struggled. I was frightened by her screams and yearned to help her. Once my sister Katie was born, my mother grew weaker after pregnancy, birth, and breastfeeding.

In May, my mother's sister our Aunt Mary visited from England to help care for our family. It was an uncertain time and my aunt role modelled to me how a strong woman can take charge and ease the pain of the hardship and misery. It was as if God had sent us an angel to watch over and care for us.

After five long gruelling months of illness and heartache, my sweet baby sister, Katie, died of tuberculosis on July 7, at only five months and twenty days old. The loss was a merciless experience. To have loved a little baby so dearly and desire to nurse and care for her, even at my young age, was almost too much to bare. I was determined to help and often resisted the doctor's orders not to go near her or my mother despite them being so sick.

Shortly after the funeral, I saw my mother fade away right before my innocent eyes. I was helpless to assist her through all the agony and misery. My mother lost weight, did not leave her bed, coughed uncontrollably as she experienced constant fever and chills.

Many expectant mothers died during this time or shortly after childbirth because of physical stress and potential infections particularly linked to tuberculosis, also known as consumption. During this era childbearing and consumption were two of the biggest threats to a woman's life and an unconscious fear that would become deeply rooted within me.

I yearned to be once again comforted by my mother, but her strength weakened, her breath shortened, and her spirit finally succumbed to silence.

16

It broke my family's hearts when our beloved mother died of consumption on October 21, 1885 in our home at 44 years of age. We buried her on October 23, next to Lillie and Katie, at Cedar Grove Cemetery in Dorchester, Massachusetts.

When I look back on the loss of my sister and mother, I am unsure if I could truly mourn their loss at five years of age, but I felt a fire inside me—a sense of injustice that grew and grew as I got older, and I knew if I ever could, I would help people who were suffering. It is therefore easy to understand how my Scottish heritage and family history influenced my lifelong dedication to my profession of helping others who were in pain and less fortunate.

My father surprised everyone by marrying Barbara Roberts, a 23-year-old housekeeper from Prince Edward Island, Canada. Her parents, Edwin and Flora Roberts, were from Canada and our family knew little history of them.

They married on July 8, 1886 in a small ceremony in Hyde Park, Massachusetts, and thus, a second McMillan family began and new siblings were added to our family. I believe that this was a common practice of the day, as so many children and childbearing mothers succumbed to illness in an era with no antibiotics on the horizon yet.

On October 11, 1886, I sailed to Liverpool at six years old because my family thought it best my Aunt Mary Livingston raise me. She was my mother's sister, and had no children of her own. They believed it would benefit me to be highly educated in England as I was only six, the only girl, and with no close siblings near my age. My brothers, Archibald (eighteen), William (thirteen), and Edward (eleven), worked in the tailor shop with my father, as it was important to our family's livelihood.

I returned to Liverpool with my aunt and met my older cousin from my mother's side, Edward William McKechnie, who lived with her and he welcomed me with open arms. We lived in a quaint

17

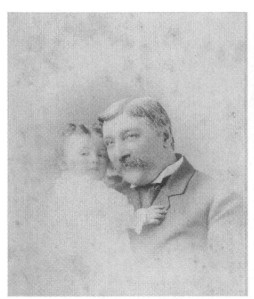
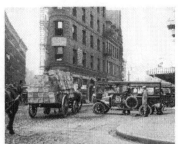
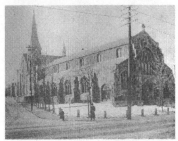
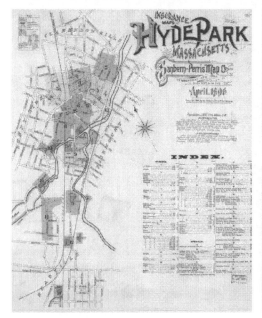
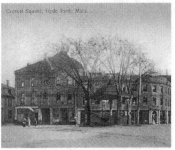
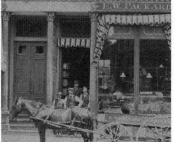

Mary's Father, Archibald McMillan and Hyde Park, Massachusetts's area where she was born

Single family home at 58 Belgrave Road in the city of Liverpool. I was delighted that the city was bustling like Boston with grand buildings that seemed to grow up out of the ground.

My Aunt Mary led me down Castle Street and to the Town Hall. It delighted me to walk across the bridge in Sefton Park and visit St. George's Hall, the Library with the Brown Museum and Picton Reading Room. She even surprised me by taking me to the Lewis department store to buy me some new clothes, which were much more in the English fashion. England was just reaching the end of the Victorian era. Three classes grew out of this period; wealthy, middle, and working poor. I believe my aunt fell into the middle of the wealthy and middle classes. I learned very quickly that etiquette was the most important distinctions between the classes. There were proper ways to walk, speak, dress, wear jewelry, how to dance, and with whom. My aunt made it clear I would be a proper lady, and I, of course, complied.

I attended the private school St. Michael's in the Hamlet during 1887 to 1900 from the ages of seven to ten years old. I settled into my new life with my aunt. I was sociable and liked meeting new friends with their wonderful British accents and dry sense of humor. December 1890 recorded as the coldest year ever and the lake froze over and my friends and I would ice skate for hours with little fear the ice would crack or break through.

During my grade school years we moved to 13 West Albert Road in St. Michael's Parish in the Hamlet near the area of Toxteth Park only a block from Sefton Park. My aunt's sister, Jeanie Gibson, came to live with us and we had one maidservant who helped my aunt cook and clean.

We often enjoyed long leisurely walks around the lake, past waterfalls, and stepping-stones. We attended church a couple times a week at St. Michael's Church in the Hamlet, a rare cast iron framed structure that had floor to ceiling stain glass. The owner of Mersey Iron Foundry, John Craig, built it in 1815 and its opening coincided with the victory celebration of the Battle of Waterloo.

19

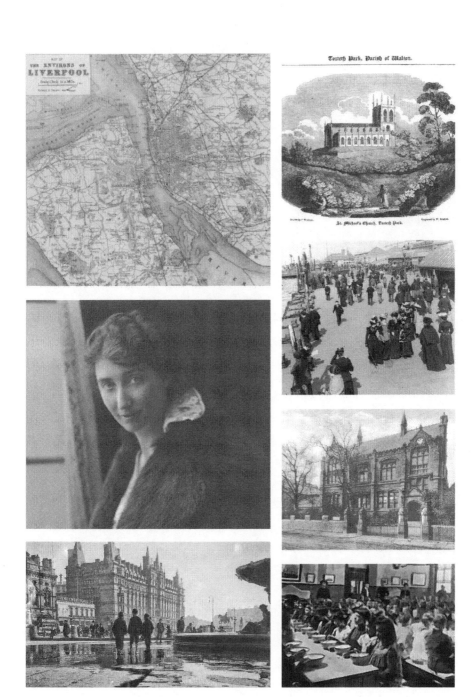

Liverpool, England: Mary in her early twenties and the Toxteth Park area where she grew up in the 1890s and 1900s

My father's new family grew quickly and my half-brother, William Edward Roberts, was born on May 21, 1889 when I was eight years old. Then my half-sister, Catherine Livingston, was born on December 2, 1890. Then two years later, my half-brother, Archibald Livingston, was brought into the world on November 28, 1892; and lastly, my half-sister, Lizzie Roberts, joined our family on May 19, 1895, the youngest of the McMillan clan who would later become my most cherished sibling.

My Boston family wrote letters often keeping connected with me while I lived far away from them. When I was eighteen years old, my Aunt Mary and I travelled on the Cephalonia Ship from Liverpool to Boston and arrived on May 7, 1889.

I spent a wonderful time with my family and it was nice to get to share this extended period with my older brothers—Archibald, John, and Edward—besides meeting my new family members, William, Catherine, Archibald Livingston, and my little sister lovey, four-year-old Lizzie.

After a two-month visit, we returned to Liverpool on the Cunard Ship Pavonia in July so that I could begin college in September. I had come to truly love and respect my dear Aunt Mary and was blessed to have been raised in her care, as I was told she was much like my mother Catherine. I received so many advantages being an only child verses growing up as one of many children in Boston, yet I was still blessed to be part of a large family of brothers and sisters who loved and cherished me within their great Scottish tribe.

It was an unhappy day when I learned of my father's death, after he died on April 25, 1900, of chronic nephritis pyelonephritis inflammation resulting from a urinary tract infection that affected his pelvis and kidneys. I felt a deep sadness, but also gratitude I had recently spent time getting to know him better before his passing.

It was a time of deep mourning for me. A period to grieve and reflect over the loss of my father, the life I might have lived with my dear McMillan family if my mother and Katie had not died, and the relationship to a family I had not been raised with but felt a deep kinship to.

21

I, Archibald Mc. Millan, of Hyde Park in the County of Norfolk and Commonwealth of Massachusetts, declare this to be my last will, hereby revoking all wills heretofore made by me.   After the payment of my just debts and funeral charges, I bequeath and devise as follows:-

1. I give to my wife, Barbara for her use for life, my dwelling house and the lands appurtenant thereto, situated on Charles Street in said Hyde Park, together with all articles of personal, domestic, or household use or ornament, including my furniture, books, pictures, provisions, consumable stores, and all household effects, which at the time of my death shall be in, about, or belonging to my said dwelling house and premises.

2. At the death of my said wife, Barbara, I devise and bequeath to my children, William E. A. Livingston, Catherine, and Elizabeth, my said dwelling house, land, and personal property above described, in equal shares, share and share alike, the child or children of any deceased child to take by right of representation.   3. I make no further provision in this will for my said wife, Barbara, inasmuch as she will receive sums of money from the various insurance policies on my life to the amount of about six thousand dollars.   It is my desire that said amount received by her as aforesaid, from my insurance policies, shall be carefully and prudently invested by her, and that the principal thereof shall go to my said children William E. A. Livingston, Catherine, and Elizabeth, at the death of my said wife Barbara,   4. In the event that my said wife Barbara, should die before me and that the said insurance policies should become payable to my estate, I bequeath the said sums of money which may be received from said insurance policies, whatever the amount thereof may be, as follows:- One-sixth thereof to my son William E. One third thereof to my son A. Livingston, One quarter thereof to my daughter Catherine, and one quarter thereof to my daughter Elizabeth.

5. I have in my lifetime given to my sons Archibald and John W. each a quarter interest in the business now carried on under the name of A. Mc. Millan + Son, at No. 127 A. Tremont Street in Boston Massachusetts, + therefore I give nothing to them in this will, except so far as they may benefit by the residuary clause hereof.   6. I bequeath to my son Edward N. and to my daughter Mary J. L. my share and interest in the said business now carried on under the name of A. Mc. Millan + Son, whatever the same may be, in equal shares, meaning and intending to bequeath hereby to my said children Edward N. and Mary J. L. all my share and interest (which now is a one-half share and interest) in the good will of said business, the stock-in-trade, fixtures, and effects belonging thereto, the benefits of all contracts subsisting in respect to said business, all book debts and moneys due to said business or standing to the credit of said business at the bank, and all and every right, title and interest in and to any property of any nature or sort whatsoever belonging to said business. My said children Edward N + Mary J. L. are to assume and discharge any and all liabilities of mine in relation to or on account of said business. My intention is that each of my children,

Mary's father, Archibald McMillan's last will and testament, 1900

2

EAGER TO LEARN

With a passion and eagerness to learn, I attended Liverpool College for Girls for two years in 1901 and 1902. It was a small school on Grove Street near the University of Liverpool. I passed junior and senior Oxford University College entrance exams.

I studied at Liverpool University—English, science, literature, French, domestic studies and hygiene in 1903 to 1905—and traveled extensively to several European countries. After two years of college, in which I was working toward a Bachelor's degree, I broke away against my family's wishes to do that—which I had wished to do more than anything else in the world.

During this time, my sisters, Kay and Lizzie, and brother, Archie Livingston, moved in with their mother's sister, Annie E. Roberts, because their mother died. Their aunt had married Francis Shutts, whose family was from New York. They had been married in Cambridge, Massachusetts, on July 25, 1888. His parents were Edgar and Annette Shutts and they lived in Chateaugay, New York, on Church Street. I wrote to them as often as I could to encourage and cheer their dear hearts.

I attended the Liverpool Gymnasium College at 171 Bedford Street from 1906 to 1908. They taught me gymnastics, physiology, hygiene, nursing, remedial exercises sports, modern games, and English, German, and Swedish massage systems with teaching credentials. I was thrilled when I earned my degree in physical education with a postgraduate degree in science.

I loved learning about physical sciences and the many ways to heal people who were suffering and knew for certain what my chosen profession was to be after graduating. Therapeutic massage was by no means a new form of therapy. Hippocrates in 460 BC used both exercise and rubbing, and in the Far East there was a book written in Chinese in 3,000 BC, called the "Cong-Fu," which dealt with prescribed manipulation movements to help people ease pain. Hippocrates and his famed teacher, Herodicus, a Greek physician, both taught gymnastics to preserve health and the cure of diseases.

Galen, a noted and respected Roman physician who lived from 130 to 200 AD, studied friction on the body and prescribed exercise to his patients. He discovered there was blood in the arteries and not air like the Greeks believed. It was not until 1628 that William Harvey discovered the circulation of the blood.

In 1770, Germans created a school for gymnastic therapy, and in 1774, Karl Adolph von Basedow expounded his ideas on exercise and the central theories based on the philosopher who lived in the 1700s, Jean-Jacques Rousseau's theory, that the body and mind assist each other in the healing process. Peter Henry Ling attended college in Germany and established the Royal Gymnastic Central Institute in Stockholm, Sweden, in 1813, and was the originator of medical gymnastics and massage. The National Health and Welfare accepted and accredited Swedish Therapists.

It thrilled me to discover that four nurses—Lucy Marianne Robinson, Rosalind Paget, Elizabeth Anne Manley, and Margaret Dora Palmer—who wanted to protect nurses from providing massage to their patients to stop unprincipled therapy practices, became active in the Chartered Society of Physiotherapy in Great Britain. In 1900, just as I began my studies, the society became incorporated for all trained massage therapists of whom I became a member.

26

I wished to learn more and discover what the United States was offering in the study of physical therapy and massage. I sailed back to America on August 19, 1906, on the ship Cymric, to spend time with my family in Boston and tour various hospitals' and doctors' offices in the East Coast area.

During this time, two Austrian physicians, Dr. Karl Landsteiner and Dr. E. Popper, identified the etiologic poliomyelitis virus in 1908. The following year, Massachusetts became the first state to count the number of poliomyelitis cases. The Polio epidemic would increase the need for more massage and rehabilitation in patients in America.

Even after all my education, I still did not believe it was enough training to do the work at the level I wanted and sought out more in-depth education on healing massage and therefore I lived in London from 1909 to 1910 to take special courses in neuroanatomy, neurology, and psychology at the Royal College of Surgeons, and also did massage and nerve work for one year.

I took Dr. Fletcher's course in scoliosis and medical gymnastics, courses on brain and spinal cord pathology at The National Hospital. Besides massage and electrotherapy in London at St. Thomas Hospital and fracture classes at London's St. George's Hospital, I studied and learned physical therapy at the Lambeth Infirmary, Massage, and Medical Gymnastics, and took my examinations and certificates from London University for Anatomy, Physiology, Medical Gymnastics, and Electrotherapy.

During this time I came to realize how much the human anatomy and physiology is linked to the whole body in a way that a magnificent orchestra plays and follows the gentle touch of a conductor's baton. All I learned never ceased to amaze me and I yearned to learn everything I could about the human body and how to ease pain and heal it.

27

I learned a great deal of information during my ten years of education and experience in the new field of physical therapy. It came intuitively to discover all I could about massage, which is derived from the Greek word to "knead" or "press." Then the word transformed into the French meaning to "manipulate body tissues." It is key to the practitioner to create energy to the areas of the body that have been exhausted or injured so the body can restore itself to its normal condition.

The body tissues influenced by massage are the skin, the fascia, the muscular system, and the nervous system. They indirectly influence the glandular, digestive, and bony systems. By reflex action through the sensory nerves in the skin, manipulation produces a sedative effect. Muscles and soft tissues are bound together by the deep superficial fascia between the layers of which are many large blood vessels.

The contraction and relaxation of the blood vessels have their beneficial effect in improving the nourishment in the cells of the entire body. Muscles are strengthened and made to grow by manipulation because it brings increased nutrition to the part the bloodstream.

Each time the muscle contraction takes place and blood forces itself through the veins, it increases the absorption of the lymph through the lymphatic vessels, accelerating the flow of arterial blood with a fresh supply of nutriment and oxygen. The motor and sensory nerves of the cerebrospinal and sympathetic systems stimulate or soothe according to the character of the manipulation used.

There are five fundamental procedures in massage that I came to understand and practice:

1. *Effleurage* is a stroking nature with the palm in two ways; first by light stroking, second by deeper stroking.

28

2. *Petrissage* is a rubbing or kneading and is performed by using the whole palm or by fingers and thumb to pick up small muscles by flexors and extensors being grasped by alternate transverse and circular moves.
3. *Friction* is manipulation in which the tips of the fingers and or thumbs around the bony prominences of joint surface bearing pressure upon underlying structures.
4. *Tapotement* is a series of brisk blows in rapid succession by hacking, clapping, tapping, or beating.
5. *Vibration* is performed with several fingers, or even with one, and at times the whole palm of the hand, a trembling sensation that conveys over the most cutaneous part of a nerve.

I felt I was now ready and prepared to begin my career in physical therapy. I returned to Liverpool in 1910 and took my first professional position working at the clinic of Sir Robert Jones, the nephew and professional heir of the great orthopedic Hugh Owen Thomas. Jones was a famed physician renowned for using the Thomas splint invented by his famous uncle and performing progressive massage and orthopedics.

29

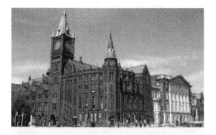

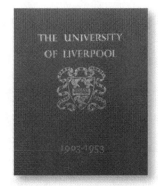

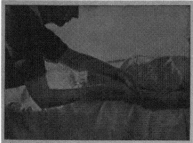

Fig. 2.—Position of hands for effleurage and petrissage of forearm.

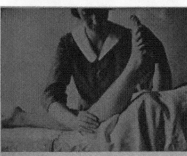

Fig. 22.—Patient in prone lying position for flexion of knee-joint if
forcible stretching is necessary in cases of fibrosis.

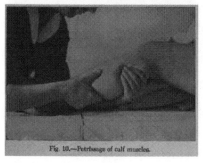

Fig. 10.—Petrissage of calf muscles.

*University of Liverpool, Mary showing examples of massage techniques and
Liverpool Gymnasium Training College advertisement*

3

FOLLOWING ONE'S PASSION

My first official job began in 1910 as an assistant to Sir Robert Jones, the General Surgeon at the Royal Southern Hospital in Liverpool. I was blessed to learn and work with the great doctor, who was a pioneer of orthopaedics and a healer, teacher of disabled people, particularly children.

Within two years they put me in charge of a children's clinic in the main hospital besides training nurses. I received a raise of £300 per year and felt as though I was truly paving the way for us to integrate physical therapy into daily practices and procedures.

I also worked part-time as a masseuse and exercise therapist at the Greenbank Cripples Rest Home on Penny Lane. Sir Robert Jones partnered with Agnes Hunt to establish the Robert Jones and Agnes Hunt Orthopaedic Hospital (RJAH) in Oswestry, in Shropshire, England in 1905 to meet the needs of children who were suffering from diseases or incurable cripples. At the time, hospitals and clinics setup to provide short-term care, and the home provided those who needed prolonged care. At first they gave me the title of Medical Gymnast and Masseuse with my first salary of £50 to 100 a year.

The Cripples Home had large rooms to accommodate the 30 kids who still enjoyed playing, even though they were disabled and ill. We even had a greenhouse that, in the winter, was a playhouse. We practiced open-air treatments and left the windows open as often as possible and took the kids outdoors. Besides medical care, the home provided them an education and religious services. In addition, we created a workshop where kids did handicrafts and sold their creations.

Sir Robert Jones became very interested in new X-ray machines after he hurt his foot dancing. They put in an X-ray machine into the new operating theatre, which was built in Baschurch to help diagnose the patients. This decision would later transform the hospital to help heal bone and joint diseases by using the X-ray machine, in addition to outside and natural sunlight used at the Cripples Home to help heal patients. The hospital would become a model for many other countries.

World War I, also known as the Great War, would test the hard work of all our efforts and put to good use all I had learned. On June 28, 1914, the war ignited after a long simmering conflict between European powers. The tipping point was the assassination of Archduke Franz Ferdinand of Austria-Hungary, who was the designated heir to the Austrian-Hungarian Empire. In a tangle of alliances, one thing led to another and Austria-Hungary declared war on Serbia and Bulgaria, Germany and the Ottoman Empire joined them as well and fought against Great Britain, France, Italy, Japan, Russia, Romania, and the United States.

In the first four years of the war, nearly nine million people died and millions more were maimed, crippled, grief stricken, and psychologically scarred—and there would be many years of healing left to all who survived. This was a tipping point for this new profession and physical therapists would become totally necessary for the rehabilitation of the wounded war survivors. A time for our work to make changes that were only dreamed of before the war.

They asked Sir Roberts Jones to become a mobilized surgeon for the Royal Army Medical Corps because of the high number of patients with broken bones. Because of his talent and skills, the British Government made him the Director of Military Orthopedics with the title Major General.

34

In 1914, the first shiploads of wounded Belgian soldiers were taken to an improvised hospital in London and Liverpool. Sir Thomas Barr oversaw all of the operations at the hospital in Liverpool. He was a surgeon-in-chief and president of the British Medical Association, which had 25,000 members.

I read the newspaper recruiting advertisements of the righteous war and suffering soldiers that I felt I must help. I had signed up for the British Army; they rejected me because of health issues as I suffered from acute tonsillitis.

In October 1914, I volunteered my services for massage work with the wounded soldiers in hospital three days a week until February 1915. I felt excluded by the British Army and discouraged because I was only given a red patch to wear to show my commitment to the cause. But what I wanted was my official gabardine uniform with the greatcoat and to be on the battlefield as so many young idealistic people of that era longed for. It was a war that needed the talents and sacrifices of so many and yet I did not realize that my real call to duty would come so much sooner than I could imagine.

I made the time to be with my dear Aunt Mary Livingston when she died on October 4, 1914. My cousin Edward and I were the benefactors of her estate; they read her will out loud to us on November 14. We were both surprised and blessed to share the effects of her estate, which they estimated at £968, which was quite a lot of money in the day. We buried her in her plot at Toxteth Park Cemetery and had her favorite quote carved in her headstone, "Until the daybreak, and the shadows flee away. A verse from Song of Solomon 4:6."

My aunt's death was a great loss to me. I never forgot how she took me into her home and heart when I was a child and was always there to nurture and listen. I was not only cared for by her but also molded to be the best Christian I could be. My Aunt Mary had

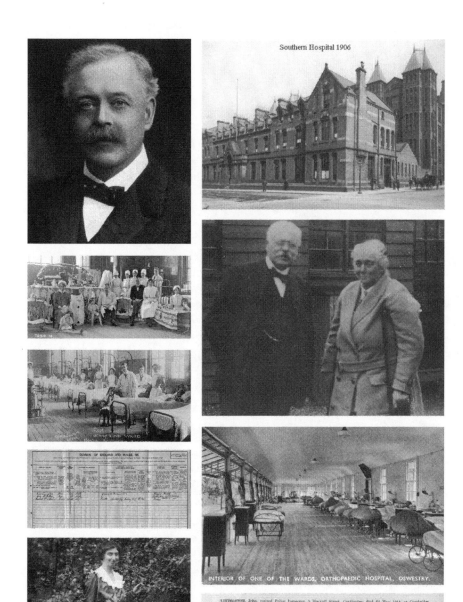

*Sir Robert Jones; Southern Hospital patients; Sir Jones and Agnes Hunt
pictured over their children's hospital ward, 1911; Mary in her mid-twenties;
her Aunt Mary Livingston's death announcement, 1914*

never held me back, not even when I was young. She role modeled for me what it was to be a strong, resilient, and self-reliant woman. As a child, I learned from the scriptures that each person has a special role in this world, and we should listen to that call. I yearned to be astute and pay attention to what my heart was telling me which was not always easy. Even though following my vocation would be difficult, especially since I was a single woman, I would now be responsible for myself and follow my own destiny wherever it lead me—and because of that, I risked it because I believed my efforts could truly make a difference in the world.

The loss of my aunt, in addition to all the soldiers dying in World War I, brought a deep sadness to my spirit, but also ignited the Scottish fight within me. I was not one to wallow in the plight of playing a victim in a great tragedy. I was a fighter and yearned to be part of something bigger than myself and the little work I was doing to help part-time with Sir Thomas Barr and the soldiers was not enough for me.

After my aunt's passing, I continued my job at the children's hospital and volunteered part-time with the wounded warriors who were suffering through the spring of 1915. My intuition kept taunting me to make a change and I wondered if my skills could be better used elsewhere. I desired to serve mankind in a more productive and powerful way.

I reflected on my purpose in life and did much soul searching. I had been considering how wonderful it would be to reunite with my family in Boston. I had been well trained, a great world war was decimating and wounded soldiers desperately needed therapy. Physicians were trying new and untested methods in the curative practices of broken bones and painful injuries. I had a rare gift and knew how to help them in the areas of anatomy, physiology, muscle movement and a myriad of healing techniques.

37

It was clear after much prayer that my unwavering passion to help those in need, my talent as a therapist was unique and could be used to help many victims of the impending battle. Simply put, I knew nothing of what the future held, but intuitively believed I was ordained to devote my life to this work and at any personal cost followed my destiny that was waiting for me in America.

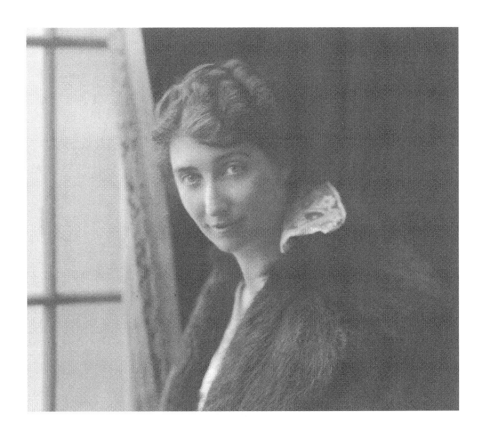

Mary McMillan in her early twenties in a photo studio

PART TWO
1916–1920

4

A LEAP OF FAITH

I sailed on the S.S. Philadelphia on July 17, 1915 from Liverpool to Boston to reunite with my family and start a new life in America. The city had thrived in the 25 years since I was born. The *Boston Chronicle* began its first publication and the city offered the citizens cherished public gardens, libraries, opera houses, grand hotels, and culture abound.

After my extended visit with my family, the Children's Hospital in Portland, Maine hired me immediately because of my education and experience. At first I worked as a "medical gymnast and masseuse," with Dr. E. G. Abbott, the doctor in charge. He truly appreciated the work I was doing and how efficient I was.

They promoted me after two years to the Director of Massage and Medical Gymnastics, treating children with scoliosis, congenital hip dislocations, and other childhood orthopaedic bone and joint abnormalities.

I also taught nurses' training classes in massage at two other hospitals in Maine. I earned an extra $300 a month at Saint Mary's Hospital in Lewiston and Webber Hospital in Biddeford.

The first major poliomyelitis epidemic happened in the summer of 1916. There were over 27,000 cases and 6,000 deaths reported in the nation with 9,000 in New York State alone. Doctors believed the best form of treatment was quarantine and isolation, but they were wrong.

The unfortunate treatment of patients was long-term splinting and casting to restrain the limbs or the spine, besides bed rest. What

43

they did not know was this regimen increased muscle weakness and lessened flexibility in the patient's extremities, which ultimately required increasing physical therapy intervention and much longer rehabilitation.

Sir Robert Jones wrote to me and sent me a copy of his new book. It was a published textbook on Orthopaedic titled *Injuries of Joints*, which explained how to deal with the diagnosis and treatment of acute fractures. When I was in London, I used to spend time in the afternoons performing practical work with fractures and dislocation. His book affirmed all I could put to good use on the wounded soldiers.

On January 2, 1917 I received a letter from Major Elliot G. Brackett recognizing the receipt of my letter dated the 29th, responding to their request if I could some way be of service. He advised me that plans were being developed for a course in intensive instruction to the United States Army Medical Aides in the work of special massage and remedial exercises in hospitals or other formations, especially for orthopaedic patients. He was not sure when he would return to Boston, but suggested I write to Miss Anderson.

There was no such profession as Physical Therapy yet when I performed massages and exercise therapy for Orthopaedic patients in the Children's Hospital. Though the profession was recognized in a few European countries, it was relatively unknown in the United States until 1917, when the Surgeon General, William C. Gorgas— just a year before he planned to retire from the Army— sent letters out to colleges and universities asking them to establish training programs to rehabilitate the vast number of wounded soldiers.

The schools chosen were, the Physical Education department of Leland Stanford University in California; the Boston School for Physical Education; the Posse Normal in Boston; the New Haven Normal School in Connecticut; the Normal School for Physical

44

Education in Battle Creek, Michigan; the Teacher's Physical Education Program at Oberlin College, Ohio; and Reed College in Portland, Oregon.

In addition, Dr. Gorgas sent several physicians to Europe to study and report on other reconstruction programs. The outcome of the account was to establish a Division of Special Hospitals and Physical Reconstruction. They investigated how people wounded in the war were being medically treated in England and France. Upon their return to the United States, they developed a plan to meet the needs of the over 200,000 United States wounded troops at the battlefront.

Their report recommended massage and mechanical hydrotherapy for patients, in addition to implementing a national training force of therapists who could provide treatments. It suggested that the personnel draw from schools of physical training and allied therapies. The board outlined standards developed by the schools that would give students the title of "physical reconstruction aides."

On April 16, 1917 the United States declared war on Germany and this ignited a major crossroads in the profession of physical therapy. The United States Army recruited women to train and assist Orthopaedic surgeons in healing physical disabilities to injured soldiers. Women signed up from all over the United States and were assigned to the newly formed Division of Special Hospitals and Physical Reconstruction in the United States Army's Office of the Surgeon General. These "reconstruction aides" served in a civilian capacity in military hospitals both in America and overseas. It established the first school of physical therapy at Walter Reed Army Hospital in Washington, DC.

At the recommendation of Sir Robert Jones and Major Elliot G. Brackett, a Boston orthopedist and one of the organizers of the Army's Reconstruction Program asked me to consider service with

45

the United States Army. I received the following telegram: *Two pioneer aides needed at Walter Reed Hospital immediately. Work, do teaching. Would you consider when you were free from present duties—am eager to get best person. Wire yes or no immediately.* Signed, *Surgeon General Gorgas.*

I was curious to find out more about how I could help the United States Army and met Mary Marguerite Sanderson at the request of Dr. Brackett, after they called him away to England. Sanderson had been doing corrective exercises in Dr. Joel Goldthwait's office, who later became the chairman of the War Reconstruction Committee for the American Orthopedic Association. The Reconstruction Committee hired Marguerite Sanderson under this new division as Director of the Reconstruction Aide Program. She had the immense task of organizing and directing all the new therapists for overseas duty. She quickly established a training program for reconstruction aides at Walter Reed General Hospital.

I knew her as being as strong as a man and undeterred by "the men on the hill." She persisted in getting the women in the army out of skirts and into pants, which was much more practical in the rain and mud.

Sanderson asked me if I wanted to help her in the Reconstructive Department of the

United States Army and on December 9, 1917, I wrote to the Surgeon General stating I was happy to accept the position. I packed my bags right away and waited for the army's official instructions.

46

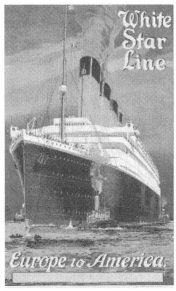
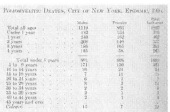
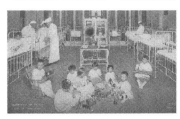
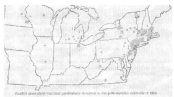
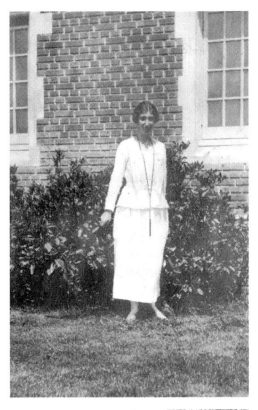
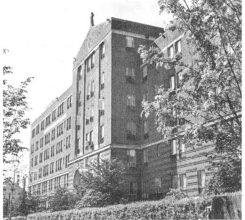

Ship Mary took to the United States, Mary in her late twenties, polio epidemic statistics, and Children's Hospital in Portland, Maine

5

FIRST EVER PHYSICAL THERAPIST SWORN INTO THE UNITED STATES ARMY

On January 2, 1918 I received a letter from the War Department office of the Surgeon General, addressed to my attention at Children's Hospital, acknowledging the letter I sent them on December 29, agreeing to instruct their Medical Aides. To my surprise, E. J. Brehaut Major stated I was to be the first recognized physical therapist in the country.

It thrilled me to receive another letter dated February 23 from the War Department Office of the Surgeon General, officially appointing me as a Reconstruction Aide in the Medical Department United States Army. Then I received another follow-up letter from Marguerite Sanderson, the Supervisor of Reconstructive Aides, on February 25, outlining the terms of my position and salary of $50 per month for my work in the Medical Department of the United States Army.

On February 23, 1918 they swore me in as a member of the United States Army Medical Corps as the first Reconstruction Aide and verbally ordered me to Walter Reed General Hospital in Takoma Park, Washington, DC. to Marguerite Sanderson, the Supervisor Reconstructive Aides.

They informed me they sent all wounded American soldiers to that hospital and I was to report directly and bring my St. John's Cross documentation, which would serve as a substitute for a certificate.

I left right away with no official orders and arrived at the Surgeon General's office where I met with Sanderson. We drove to Walter Reed Hospital, which was only six miles from the White House. Sanderson personally escorted me through Walter Reed Hospital. It was a vast medical building built ten years earlier. They designed the main administration building in a Colonial Georgia Revival style, which was at the center of the property.

After my tour I walked to the recently built Army School of Nurses, where over 400 newly trained nurses were bustling around the building and grounds. Then we passed along the tree-lined walkway by the barracks located on the side main building. I began the next day working at Walter Reed Hospital in Washington, DC. as the Director of Special Courses with an increase of salary to $250 a month with board extra. In March, they promoted me to the Head Reconstruction Aide and I was feeling like I was truly making a difference.

I was new to the army and had no idea how things were to run, but learned quickly. The hospital only had a small hydrotherapy department in the basement but it was well run. I remembered thinking this was a poignant moment in American History as it was the inception of physical therapy in the United States Army.

There was no place for me to work in, except the small basement with a couple of hydrotherapy tubs, so I asked for an area to set up a new Physical Therapy department and they unenthusiastically replied that they would consider it. No one at the hospital knew what physical therapy was and I had to "sell" this new healing technique and myself to the doctors and patients. It was a tough sell because the Walter Reed doctors had little time or interest in the likes of me.

I decided that I needed to make a sort of calling card for the doctors to use to direct their patients to me, so I had some prescription forms printed up and took them around the hospital as if selling encyclopaedias door-to-door. I told the doctors and nurses to fill out the forms as if they were prescribing the work I was doing just like medicine. I encouraged them to send their suffering patients my way. I assured them I could ease their pain.

At first they were reluctant and skeptical, as if I was a snake salesman selling my secret potions that would somehow cure their patients. They did not believe massage, hydrotherapy and nurturing one's spirit that they would soon feel better would make a difference in their patient's healing.

I knew I would need to use my good humor, Scottish charm, and determination to win these doctors over. They thought I was a bit of an intruder and doubtful of the treatments. In a couple cases, doctors even warned their patients not to trust me, as I might do more damage than good.

There were two doctors who finally took notice of my work and became curious about my efforts and exertion. Dr. Frederic J. Cotton U.S. Army was a great surgeon who had been promoted to the Therapy Department. He had a keen interest and constructive criticism how we could do things better, which I was always open and eager to learn about the techniques I doing.

Dr. Cotton was from Boston and had invented an anaesthesia apparatus in 1911 with his colleague Dr. Walter Boothby at Boston City Hospital. It helped to provide uninterrupted flow of oxygen through the chambers to help the gauge how to add ether vapour to the gas mixture.

My other convert was Dr. Frank B. Granger of Harvard Medical School who headed our new department. He became the biggest advocate of the work we were doing. He was conservative in manner, yet progressive in spirit.

And finally the Surgeon General agreed with the Dr. Granger's opinion and wrote that our department showed continence, which would help the first reconstruction aides to establish our new kind of vocation.

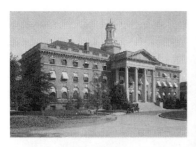
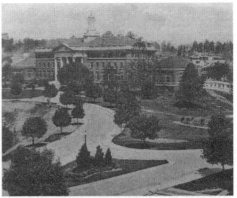
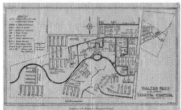
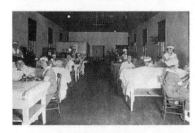
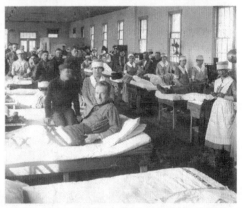
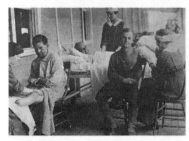
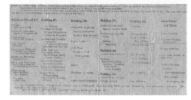
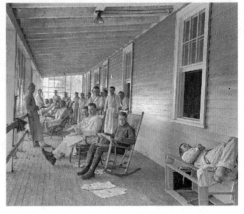

*Walter Reed Hospital, United States Army's flagship medical center
in Washington, DC, and wounded soldiers*

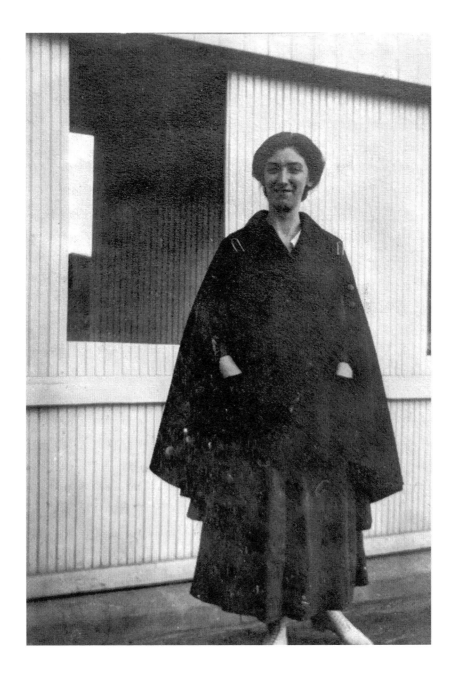

Mary McMillan sworn in as the first Reconstruction Aide of the United States Army Medical Corps on February 23, 1918

ALL ARMY HOSPITALS TO GIVE PHYSIO-THERAPY TREATMENT

Methods Developed by Capt. Charles L. Ireland at Walter Reed, Which Sends Out 100 Physicians as Surgeons.

DOING A GREAT WORK AT WALTER REED

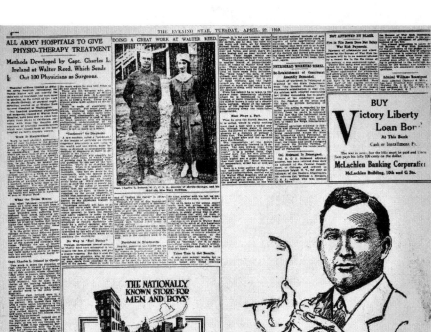

Capt. Charles L. Ireland, M. C., U. S. A., director of physio-therapy, and his chief aid, Miss Mary McMillIan.

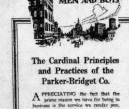

Noted for Cheerfulness.

Dr. Ireland—or Capt. Ireland, as he is known now—is one of the very cheeriest persons in the great ward which is noted for that very quality. Cheerfulness forms part of the treatment. While the business of those in charge is to build up the physical conditions of the men, the far-reaching results of mental suggestion are not forgotten.

That is one reason why this ward has about the prettiest corps of nurses to be found anywhere. These forty-five girls, in their blue uniforms, are believed by some to be the prettiest girls at Walter Reed. They all are college graduates, women of high standards, who are experts in their line.

Miss Mary McMillan is chief of aids. Miss McMillan originated the work at Walter Reed and was later sent to various posts throughout the country to put in operation at the other hospitals the system used at the local hospital. She was brought back to Walter Reed Hospital the first of the present month.

They decided that Marguerite Sanderson would oversee all the reconstruction aides in the Division of Physical Reconstruction, and I would organize and manage the operations at the hospital. Then, to my surprise on March 5, 1918, I received a letter from Sanderson at the War Department Office of the Surgeon General promoting me to the Head of Reconstruction Aides of the United States Army and that my oath of office should be taken, if possible, on that day before a notary public and mailed back to the enclosed envelope. On March 9, I received my official promotion letter.

I was alone at the hospital for a few weeks and found myself in the basement with little equipment and small hydrotherapy section. There was no treatment space or equipment for me to work with, so at first I spent most of my time giving bedside treatments of massage and hot fomentations. Finally the doctors and patients began to see a difference and I was given the sun porch area to provide therapy sessions.

Igna Lohne, a Norwegian expatriate, was the next aide to arrive. They swore her in as second Physical Reconstruction Aide to the United States Army. She was an excellent worker—earnest and efficient—always full of spirit and enthusiasm. Then, Inga Lohne Brauner joined as the third of the group of eighteen women who were to be included in the first elite company of reconstruction aides. She was from Norway and moved to America to attend Teachers College at Columbia University. After graduating she traveled throughout Europe and visited gymnasiums in Scandinavia and other countries during 1915 and 1916. She returned to the United States to volunteer her services during World War I.

Next to join our group were Helen Sheddon, Margery Rickok, Josephine Bell, and Dorothea Beck. After their training, Hazel Furscott was assigned to Fort McPherson, Georgia; Beck would become the Head of Reconstructive Aides in Texas; Rickok and Bell worked at Letterman's Hospital in San Francisco; and Constance.

56

Green served with the United States Army in France, while Marguerite Irvine devoted her professional career to the Army. And thus the inaugural group of women began the new profession of physical therapy, with eighteen keen and ardent reconstruction aides who had a sincere passion to help others.

Our physical therapy hospital staff gave 5,000 treatments a week and the number increased to 8,000 a week—helping a total of 25,000 patients. We began using a new machine, a "condenser" that, when applied to the muscle, automatically releases a current and stimulates the nerves, which is recorded on a reflex chart. In addition, the nurses used their healing hands and skill to help build and strengthen the soldiers' muscles.

While I served at Walter Reed Hospital, I attended Dr. R. W. Lovett Special six-week Orthopedic Course in Washington, DC. I had learned early in the study of physical therapy that while the human body does not change, the ways and inventions on how to heal and repair the body evolves and grows, and it is a complex puzzle yet to be solved.

One day we heard rumors we might get our own physical therapy building, and indeed we did. Dr. Granger equipped the building with the much-needed equipment and we gave courses to our new reconstruction aides. It was a large U-shaped building with a pool in the middle of it. There were a couple dozen-treatment rooms, a gymnasium, and special equipment sections. I was excited and enthusiastic to work with the director of the department, Major T. M. McFee and was determined to establish a high set of standards and lay a strong foundation for this new profession.

On June 6, 1918, Sanderson saw the first organization and reconstruction aides off to Europe to begin their specialized duties to physically rehabilitate individuals who would be wounded on the battlefield. They did such a great job spreading the organization's mission; our reputation grew with both doctors and patients.

On June 18, 1918 the National Society of Reconstruction Work held an all day conference in Baltimore at Fort McHenry Hospital, to discuss the entry of homeopathic practitioners in the Medical Reserve Corps, division of physical therapeutics. Dr. Granger shared he could use all the physical therapist that would apply. He ordered and approved 40 Reconstruction Hospitals to set up around the country and to provide Electrotherapy, Hydrotherapy, Massage, Mechanotherapy and Medical Exercise.

At the time, the Baltimore hospital was the only reconstruction therapy unit near its completion. Granger toured the hospital with the other doctors. Col. Frank S. Billings of Chicago had been put in charge of the entire Reconstruction work and Granger the head of the physical therapeutics division.

At this time I split my time, mornings at Walter Reed Hospital and the afternoons at the Surgeon General's office looking after the emergency hospitals that were closing and juggling where patients needed to go. I also took an electrotherapy class for six weeks, two hours per week with Dr. Baker.

In the fall of 1918, the Surgeon General, Merritte W. Ireland, MD of the Medical Department of the United States Army, created two divisions that induced the development of physical therapy. The first was the Division of Physical Reconstruction and the second, the Division of Orthopedic Surgery. Ireland was one of the most inspiring doctors I worked work with; his compassionate heart and bright smile healed the wounded hearts and bodies.

All wounded soldiers in the United States would eventually experience all the same treatment because of the work and teaching carried out at Walter Reed Hospital and overseen by Ireland. The physiotherapy department set up a protocol and directed using forms of electricity and massage to loosen stiffened body, legs, and arms to release toxins.

58

In addition, prominent orthopedic doctors from Boston—Elliott G. Brackett, MD; Joel E. Goldthwaite, MD; Frank B. Granger, MD; and Marguerite Sanderson—who had graduated from the Boston Normal School of Gymnastics and had been working with Goldthwaite joined the Division of Orthopedic Surgery, which called for the establishment of hospitals for the reconstruction of soldiers with disabilities. They organized and developed the official Reconstruction Aide Program.

The new Division of Physical Reconstruction set up and headed by Joel Goldthwaite, M.D., had been the first Chief of Orthopedics at Massachusetts General Hospital from 1904 to 1911. He became the Chairman of the War Reconstruction Committee of the American Orthopedic Association, and Frank Granger, MD was the director of Physiotherapy of Service of Reconstruction Division.

59

DRAFT "B"   THE AMERICAN RED CROSS
NATIONAL HEADQUARTERS
WASHINGTON, D. C.

INTER-OFFICE LETTER

To   All Division Directors of Civilian Relief   Date   August 6, 1918.

From   Director General of Civilian Relief

Subject   Reconstruction Aides.

1. Referring to B-238, one of the Division offices inquired whether it would not be possible to obtain some further idea of the plans of the Surgeon General's Office in order to answer inquiries which are constantly received as to the number of women who are likely to be required for service as reconstruction aides and as to the prerequisites of education, special training in nursing, craft work, age, etc., required of those who wish to undertake this work.

2. These questions were referred to Colonel Frank Billings, Chief of the Division of Reconstruction of the Surgeon General's Office, who has replied as follows:

"It is impossible to state at this time just how many Reconstruction Aides in Occupational Therapy the Medical Department of the Army may need during the next year ending June 30, 1919. The American Red Cross furnishes the Reconstruction Aides for service overseas their military uniforms and necessary equipment. We have indicated to the American Red Cross that there will probably be a need overseas of two hundred Reconstruction Aides during the next year. Of these, one hundred approximately, will be Reconstruction Aides in Occupational Therapy. In the general hospitals of the United States which function in physical reconstruction of disabled soldiers, we will utilize some of these Reconstruction Aides probably where needed in the proportion of one to twenty-five disabled soldiers. In the hospitals of one thousand beds, handcrafts will be needed in the wards for approximately two hundred men, or in other words there will be a need of approximately eight Reconstruction Aides in Occupational Therapy for a hospital of one thousand beds. We estimate that we will have under treatment in the general military hospitals of this country during the next year approximately twenty thousand disabled soldiers. Approximately we will need two hundred Reconstruction Aides in Occupational Therapy to meet our need in the United States during the next year.

The pre-requisites as to age fixed for the present is healthy women from twenty-five to forty years of age. If the Reconstruction Aide in Occupational Therapy is utilized in the hospitals of this country she may be a married woman and may be the wife of an officer of the army. If her husband is overseas she could not be sent overseas under the ruling of the War Department. They must of course be citizens of the United States, physically they must be fit, should not be less than sixty inches in height nor more than seventy inches. They should weigh not less than one hundred nor more than one hundred ninety-five pounds.

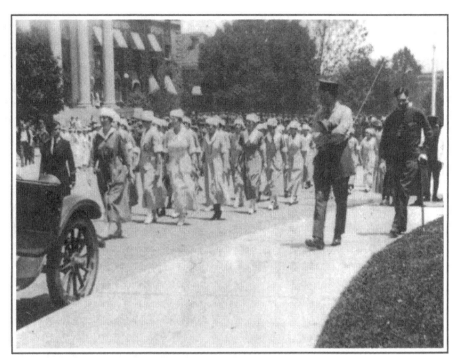

Mary McMillan in dark dress at the head of her "reconstruction aides"
Walter Reed General Hospital, 1919. (Armed Forces Institute of Pathology)

and oversaw all of the training programs. Then the government put out a call for 20,000 additional nurses due to the hundreds of thousands of soldiers that would suffer and be wounded in battle.

The division had three special sections. The first was education, which handled physiotherapy, including equipment, gymnasiums, and other edifices. The second was the clinical work, which included general surgery, orthopedic surgery, head surgery, and neuropsychiatry; and the third was the actual physical therapy practices in which clinicians prescribed certain types therapy services carried out by the reconstruction aides.

Their plan was to create two different groups of aides. One group was to assist the physicians, and were titled reconstruction

61

aides and physical therapists. These were to provide exercise programs, hydrotherapy and other modalities, and massage for these patients. The other group was providing the training in the vocational skills of the day needed for patients to cope, manage, and return to gainful employment.

In 1918, Sanderson delivered a speech entitled, "The Massage Problem," expressing her concern that doctors, nurses, and patients alike might construe therapeutic massage as "medically dubious" at best and elicit at worst. The aides sought to address this challenge by requiring professional physiotherapy education, treating only those who were medically in need of care and "assuming command of drill and sporting events," in which the women played against the soldiers.

Besides learning different physical therapy techniques, therapists often confronted some unique challenges providing care to male soldiers. The aides were required to be trained in military style marching and drills before going off to war. They quickly opened emergency hospitals and Dr. Everett Breach at Reed College called me to tell me 200 girls were waiting for training and asked if I would come. The United States Army was in desperate need for "war reconstruction aides" and in order to meet the needs of patients, we needed to train them quickly. I told him, "I will go wherever you think the best place I can be of service."

It took a lot of back and forth with my commanding officers, but I finally got my leave of absence from the army in June 1918, at the urgent request of the president of Reed College. The Surgeon General finally granted me official leave from Walter Reed General Hospital. I happily accepted the position of Director of Reconstruction Aides to train two emergency classes of physiotherapists at Reed College in Portland, Oregon.

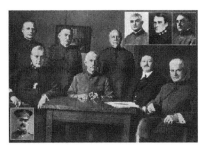

Executive Committee of the General Medical Board: (standing) Frank F. Simpson, Victor C. Vaughan, William H. Welch; (upper inset) William J. Mayo, Cary T. Grayson, Charles H. Mayo; (seated) Surgeon General (USN) William C. Braisted, Surgeon General (Army) William C. Gorgas, Surgeon General (USPHS) Rupert Blue, Franklin H. Martin; (lower inset) Jefferson R. Kean

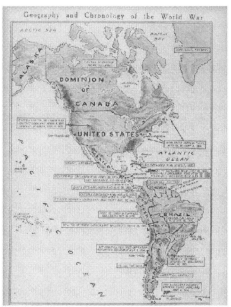

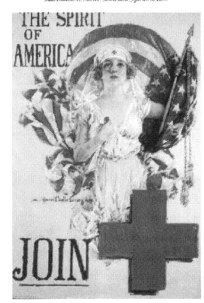

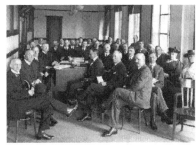

Committee on Standardization

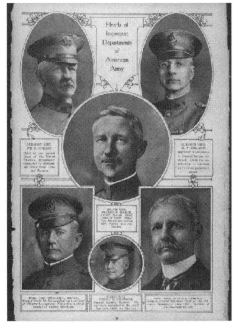

World War key leaders with geography and chronology maps

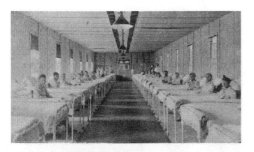

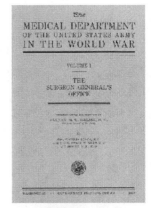

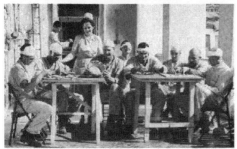

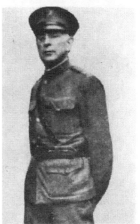

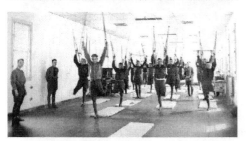

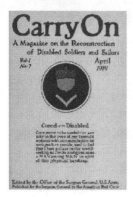

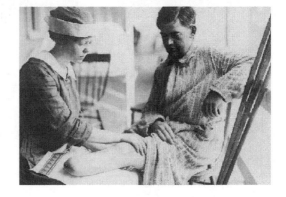

Walter Reed Hospital, Major Elliot G. Brackett, wounded soldiers, and Carry On Magazine

Where Can a Woman Serve?

A Big Field is Open for Reconstruction Aides

By Major M. E. Haggerty, S. C., U. S. A.

As the war goes on the women of America show an increasing desire to help in all fields of service—at home and overseas. Interest in the handicapped soldier and sailor is especially sharp, and thousands of women seek definite information from the Government as to how they can devote their time and experience to the work of reconstruction.

Our men are returning in large numbers and there is immediate need in military hospitals for trained women to act as Reconstruction Aides. Approximately 2,000 such women will be needed for overseas service within the next few months, others at home. Reconstruction Aides are divided into groups: Physio-Therapy and Occupational Therapy.

In Physio-Therapy they are required to have a minimum general education equivalent to graduation from a graded school. Their professional training consists in theoretical and practical knowledge in Physio-Therapy embracing Hydro-Therapy, Electro-Therapy, Mechano-Therapy, and Massage. Each aide must be qualified in at least two of these specialized branches.

Reconstruction Aides in Occupational Therapy are teachers of handcrafts and other subjects to disabled soldiers in military hospitals. They are required to have a general education, at least the equivalent to graduation from a secondary school. Normal school and college graduates and those with comparable technical training will be preferred. Applicants for Reconstruction Aides in Occupational Therapy should be capable of giving service as follows:

Class A. Expert in one or more lines in this class. (Some experience as a teacher is desired, but not required.)

Social worker

Library service

Teacher of adolescents or adults in

       Industrial and fine arts

       General science

       English

       Commercial branches

       Free-hand drawing and design

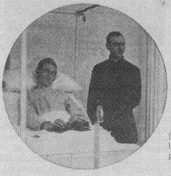

Learning telegraphy in bed—an example of practical curative work.

(#10121)

WAR DEPARTMENT
Office of the Surgeon General.
Washington.

February 23, 1918.

WITH THE APPROVAL OF THE SECRETARY OF WAR.

Miss Mary McMillan
of Portland, Maine,
is hereby appointed Reconstruction Aide, United States Army, Medical
Department, at large, at $50.00 per month with rations and lodging and
enter upon her duties after taking the oath prescribed by section
1757 of Revised Statutes of the United States.

W.C.GORGAS

Surgeon General, U. S. Army,

By (sgd)   ?

Colonel Medical Corps

855

Oath taken 2/26/18.

COPY.

(COPY SENT TO NURSES QUARTERS)

WAR DEPARTMENT
OFFICE OF THE SURGEON GENERAL
WASHINGTON

February 25, 1918.

From: The Surgeon General, U. S. Army,

To: Miss Mary McMillan, 502 S. 49th. Street, Philadelphia, Pa.

Subject: Appointment, Reconstruction Aide, Medical Department, U.S.Army.

1. I am directed by the Surgeon General to inform you that you
have been appointed a Reconstruction Aide in the Medical Department, U.S.
Army, and that you are by the terms of your appointment to enter upon your
duties thereunder after taking the Oath of office, blank therefor enclosed
herewith.

2. The Oath should be executed not earlier than the 25th. inst., but
if possible on that day before a notary public or other official authorized
to administer oaths, and should thereupon be mailed at once to this office
in the inclosed envelope. It is important that this Oath be properly executed in all respects; otherwise, complications may arise respecting your right
to pay and travel allowances.

3. I inclose your travel order and requests for transportation. Com-
plying with the former you will proceed without delay after having taken
the Oath to the Walter Reed General Hospital, Tacoma Park, Washington, D.C.,
and present the order to the Commanding Officer who will assign you to duty.
Tickets and Pullman car accommodations will be furnished on presentation of
the transportation requests at the railroad ticket office in your city. It
is suggested that you make your reservation for Pullman car accommodation as
soon as possible, but under no circumstances should you exchange the transportation requests for tickets or begin your journey under these travel orders
UNTIL AFTER YOU HAVE PROPERLY EXECUTED THE OATH OF OFFICE.

4. Upon receipt of the Oath by this office, your appointment will be
mailed to you to Walter Reed General Hospital, Tacoma Park, Washington, D.C.

By order of the Surgeon General:

Marguerite Sanderson
Supervisor, Reconstruction
Aides.   per E. H.

4 encls

WAR DEPARTMENT
OFFICE OF THE SURGEON GENERAL
WASHINGTON

March 5th., 1918.

From: The Surgeon General, U. S. Army,

To: Miss Mary McMillan, Reconstruction Aide, (thru Command-
         ing Officer,) Walter Reed General Hospital,Takoma Park,D.C.

Subject: Promotion to grade of Head Reconstruction Aides.

1.   The Surgeon General directs me to inform you that you have
been promoted from the grade of Reconstruction Aide to the grade of
Head Reconstruction Aide, United States Army, Medical Department, and
that you are by the terms of your promotion to enter upon your duties
thereunder after taking the Oath of office, blank therefor enclosed
herewith.

2.   The Oath should be executed not earlier than March 5th.,
but if possible on that day, before a notary public, or other public
official authorized to administer oaths, and should thereupon be mailed at once to this office in the enclosed envelope. It is important
that this Oath be properly executed in all respects, otherwise complications may arise respecting your right to pay and travel allowances.

3.   Upon receipt of the Oath by this office, your promotion will
be mailed to you to Walter Reed General Hospital, Takoma Park, D. C.

By direction of the Surgeon General:

encl 2

Supervisor, Reconstruction Aides.

1st ind.   jpk
Hq., Walter Reed General Hospital, Takoma Park, D. C., March 6, 1918.
To Miss Mary McMillan, Reconstruction Aide, Ward "A", W. R. G. H.

1.   Forwarded.

WILLARD F. TRUBY
Colonel, Medical Corps, U.S.Army.
Commanding.

ALL COMMUNICATIONS SHOULD BE ADDRESSED TO "THE SURGEON GENERAL, U. S. ARMY, WASHINGTON, D. C."

WAR DEPARTMENT
OFFICE OF THE SURGEON GENERAL
WASHINGTON

March 9, 1918.

From: The Surgeon General, U. S. Army,

To: Miss Mary McMillan, Head Reconstruction Aide, (thru the
          Commanding Officer,) Walter Reed General Hospital, Takoma
          Park, D. C.

Subject: Promotion to grade of Head Reconstruction Aide, Medical
          Department, U. S. Army.

   1.   Enclosed herewith is promotion from the grade of Reconstruction Aide to that of Head Reconstruction Aide.

   2.   Your Oath of Office was received and filed this date.

     By direction of the Surgeon General:

Marguerite Sanderson (A.N.)

              Supervisor, Reconstruction
encl   Aides.

                     1st ind.   jpk
Hq., Walter Reed General Hospital, Takoma Park, D. C., March 11, 1918.
To Miss Mary McMillan, Head Reconstruction Aide, Ward "A", W.R.G.H.

   1.   Forwarded.

Willard F. Truby

              WILLARD F. TRUBY
          Colonel, Medical Corps, U. S. Army,
                Commanding.

with the

7333

WAR DEPARTMENT

Office of the Surgeon General,

Washington.

MARY Mc MILLAN

MAY 18, 1918

WITH THE APPROVAL OF THE SECRETARY OF WAR,

MARY McMILLAN of PORTLAND, MAINE,

is hereby appointed Reconstruction Aide in the Medical Department of
the Army, at $50 a month except as hereinbelow otherwise provided, and
will enter upon her duties after having taken the oath of office prescribed by section 1757 of the Revised Statutes of the United States.

When practicable she will be furnished lodgings at the hospital
where she is serving, and in that event the commanding officer of the
hospital will receive one ration a day in her behalf and provide her
with proper meals.

When serving at a hospital where it it not practicable to lodge her
she will receive additional pay at the rate of $62.50 a month.

When serving beyond seas she will receive additional pay at the rate
of $10 a month from the time of leaving home port under orders to the time
of arriving back at home port under orders.

When designated as Head Aide she will receive additional pay at the
rate of $15 a month.

Her uniforms soiled while on public duty will be laundered as a part
of the hospital laundry.

She will receive transportation, and $4 a day in lieu of
station of duty; (b) when traveling under orders between stations of
duty; (c) when traveling under orders on return home from last station
of duty.

She will be provided with suitable lodgings and subsistence at the
cost of the United States while detained under orders at a port of em-
barkation awaiting transportation.

W. C. GORGAS

Surgeon General, U. S. Army

Carl R. Darnall
Colonel, Medical Corps

esignated as Head Reconstruction
Aide on March ., 1918, while
serving under appointment of
February 25, 1918.

By authority of the Surgeon
General:

[signature]
Colonel, Medical Corps

Walter Reed General Hospital
Takoma Park, D. C.
Reported for duty at this Hospi-
tal February 23, 1918, per Order
No. 3., N. G. O. dated February 23,
1918.
Previous service February 25,
May 17, 1918.

[signature]
Colonel, Medical Corps, U.S.A.
Commanding.

Walter Reed General Hospital
Takoma Park, D.C.
From present for duty to reserve
leave for eighty-three (83)
with pay and allowance per pp.2
from June 15, to September
1918, inclusive.

Willard F. Truby [signature]
Colonel, Medical Corps, U.S.A.
Commanding.

Walter Reed General Hospital
Takoma Park, D.C.
Last paid to include May 31, 1918.

[signature]
Lieut. Colonel, U.S.A. Retired.

Walter Reed General Hospital,
Takoma Park, D.C.
Leave of absence as granted for (83)
eighty-three days without pay or
allowance is extended to January 2
1919 per Ind. W.R.G.H. dated
August 22, 1918.

[signature]
Lt. Colonel, Medical Corps, U.S.Army,
Retired.

Walter Reed General Hospital
Takoma Park, D.C.
From absence with leave as above
granted to present for duty Jan.
30, 1919. relinquishing 2 days .

C. A. Egan [signature]
Lieut. Colonel, U.S.Army Retired.

Walter Reed General Hospital
Takoma Park, D.C.
Left this Hospital February 11, 1919
to proceed to U.S.A. General Hosp.
24, Parkview, Pa. reporting on
arrival to the Commanding Officer
for assignment to duty per S.O.
37 pp 1 W.R.G.H. dated Feb.5,
1919.
Last paid to include May 31, 1918.

C. A. Egan [signature]
Lieut. Colonel, U.S.Army Retired.

[Hospital No. —]
[— Branch, Pittsburgh,]
[Reported for temporary duty at]
[— Reed General Hospital, Tak-]
[Takoma Park D.C.]

[signature]

U. S. General Army Hospital, # 24
Parkview Station, Pittsburgh, Pa.
March 12, 1919
Report Mar McMillan, from duty to
sick at home, March 7, 1919.

E. D. Kremers
Lt. Col. Med. Corps, Commanding

U. S. General Hospital, # 24
Parkview Station, Pittsburgh, Pa.
March 12, 1919.
Report Mary McMillan, from sick
at home to sick in hospital,
March 10, 1919.

E. D. Kremers,
Lt. Col. Med. Corps, Commanding

US GH 24, Parkview, Pittsburgh, Pa.
From sick in hospital to duty
March 17, 1919.

E D Kremers [signature]
Liout. Col. Med Corps, Commanding.

US GH 24, Parkview Sta. Pittsburgh,
Pa., April 5, 1919.
Left this date for Walter Reed GH.
Takoma Park, D.C. for duty pp 2 SO
132, USGH 24, Apr 2, 1919. Last pd.
to March 31, 1919 by Lt Marcus QMC.

E D Kremers [signature]
Lieut Colonel, Medical Corps
Commanding.

EDVILLE G. ABBOTT, M. D.
HAROLD A. PINGREE, M. D.
FRANK W. LAMB, M. D.
EDWIN W. GEHRING, M. D.
THOMAS A. FOSTER, M.

Y. M. C. A. Building,
Portland, Maine.

OFFICE HOURS, 1.30 TO 3.30,
EXCEPT SUNDAYS

PATIENTS SEEN AT OTHER TIMES
BY APPOINTMENT ONLY.

July 30, 1918.

Miss Mary McMillan
Lewis Home Nineteenth and Glisan Streets
Portland, Oregon

Dear Miss McMillan:-

I am very much pleased with the "write up" of
your work in your new location. Of course I would much prefer
that you were doing the same thing in Portland, Maine, but if
we cannot have your efficiency I am glad that someone can and that
you are appreciated. We miss your directing hand at the Children's
Hospital and our work there has suffered from the loss of your
supervision. I am still strongly convinced, as I have repeatedly
told you of your special adaptation to this work, that you will
have a great future and while we deplore our loss we extend
congratulations to others who receive the benefits and apparently
appreciate your devotion to the cause. Nine out of the thirteen
men on the active staff have entered the service. I should be there
myself, I think, but have felt it my duty so far to keep on with
my work at the hospital. If, however, a few more should think it
best to leave us for what "out-siders" consider more patriotic
work it would be impossible to continue and I would be free to
follow the strongest inclination that I have ever had, namely to
give my services to a cause, which is so paramount in its
importance, that all else is not worthy of consideration.

EDVILLE G. ABBOTT, M. D.
HAROLD A. PINGREE, M. O.
FRANK W. LAMB, M. D.
EDWIN W. GEHRING, M. D.
THOMAS A. FOSTER, M. -

310
Y. M. C. A. Building,
Portland, Maine.

OFFICE HOURS, 1:30 TO 3:30.
EXCEPT SUNDAYS.

PATIENTS SEEN AT OTHER TIMES
BY APPOINTMENT ONLY.

I do hope that you have already met Pres. Foster of Reed who

perhaps has been more of an incentive for good work in my

life than any other single factor. He is so able and has such

a keen perspective of everything worth while that instead of the

"kaiser" being of Divine origin or rather in league with God I

have thought that he was. I am writing somewhat at length in

acknowledging my receipt of the newspaper clipping but you

know that I am extremely interested in what you are doing and

I want you to know that we all appreciate your work in Portland,

Maine, and also that your success is not more than we had

anticipated. If there is anything we can do to help you we

would consider it not only a duty but also a great pleasure

to lend our assistance.

Sincerely yours,

E G Abbott MD

EGA/AF

REED COLLEGE

PORTLAND, OREGON

20 August 1918

Dear Miss McMillan:

    I have tried in every way to make it clear to you
that every body connected with Reed College is eager to have you
remain with us. I take this opportunity to supplement what I
have said, and what Mr. Beach has said, with this letter, in order
that there may be no possible misunderstanding. Every body connected with the institution likes you, respects you and trusts
your leadership. We are disposed to adopt every feasible suggestion you may make. We are eager to make conditions such
that you can accomplish the greatest possible amount of good
under conditions which release your energies and make you as
happy as possible. We believe that because there is no other
woman in the entire west with your professional preparation,
your position of leadership is unique and your opportunity for
servis is larger than it would be in the east, unless something
much larger than we know about turns up, in which case we should,
of course, release you, since our interests are as broad as yours.

    I hope that you will agree to stay with us at least
until the first of January 1919; but if you prefer, we shall be
glad to have you agree to stay until the Government has a large work
entirely redy for you at San Francisco or elsewhere.

    We shall be glad to pay you two hundred dollars a
month in addition to the expenses of your room and board. We
shall be glad to arrange for you to have a vacation before the
beginning of the college here, on October first.

    Knowing your attitude toward your work, I have
held out to you as an inducement nothing but the opportunity for
servis, and my assurance that we would do everything possible
to increase that opportunity. I should call to see you again
and tell you again of my personal satisfaction in working with you
and try to persuade you to remain with us, were it not that you
rightly regard these personal considerations as of minor account.
My hope is that you will see the work with us for the present
as your largest field for doing good.

    Faithfully yours,

    William T. Foster

Miss McMillan
Reed College

CLASS OF SERVICE DESIRED

Fast Day Message	
Day Letter	
Night Message	
Night Letter	X

Patrons should mark an X oppo-
site the class of service desired;
OTHERWISE THE TELEGRAM
WILL BE TRANSMITTED AS A
FAST DAY MESSAGE.

Form 1207

WESTERN UNION
TELEGRAM

NEWCOMB CARLTON, PRESIDENT   GEORGE W. E. ATKINS, FIRST VICE-PRESIDENT

Receiver's No.

OPR. ANTHONY
Check

G.R.
Time Filed

10:15 A.M.

Send the following telegram, subject to the terms
on back hereof, which are hereby agreed to

PORTLAND OREGON, AUGUST 22-1918   191

To COLONEL TRUBY, COMMANDING OFFICER.

Street and No. WALTER REED GENERAL HOSPITAL TAKOMA PARK D.C.

Place

WE URGE YOU TO EXTEND LEAVE OF ABSENCE OF MARY MCMILLAN UNTIL JANUARY NINETEENTH
SHE IS ONLY WOMAN ON PACIFIC COAST COMPETENT TO TRAIN AIDES IN MASSAGE FOR MILITARY
HOSPITAL HAS WORKED WELL STARTED WITH TWO HUNDRED AND CAREFULLY SELECTED WOMEN AND
NOW IN TRAINING AND NEW RECONSTRUCTION CLINIC JUST OPENED MISS MCMILLAN IN FULL CHARGE
TO CONSOLIDATE HER ACHIEVEMENTS SHE SHOULD REMAIN SEVERAL MONTHS AND NOT LEAVE AT THIS
CRITICAL PERIOD SURGEON GENERAL TODAY NOTIFIES US TO SEND ENTIRE LIST OF CANDIDATES
AND EXPRESSES OF PROBABLE NEEDS OF FIFTEEN HUNDRED MORE MISS MCMILLAN IS ABSOLUTELY
ESSENTIAL FOR THIS WORK.

(SGD) W.T.FOSTER.

PRESIDENT REED COLLEGE.

SENDER'S ADDRESS
FOR ANSWER

SENDER'S TELE-
PHONE NUMBER

6

THE MOTHER OF PHYSICAL THERAPY

In June 1918, I found 208 ladies waiting for me at Reed College. This was the largest enrolment class assembled out of the seven chosen university Physical Therapy programs. These courageous women represented 72 universities or colleges from 31 states.

The summer school program had been approved by the Red Cross and they had carefully selected this group of women from the ages of 25 to 40 years, with a majority of them already having college degrees.

The students were trained in Anatomy, Aspects of Recovery, Bandaging, Military Hospital Management, Massage, Orthopedic Surgery, Personal Hygiene, Physiology, Posture, Recovery, and Remedial Exercise.

Most reconstructive aides earned their certificates during a nine-month training program. This included 240 hours of hospital experience and four months of practical and theoretical physiotherapy. But this first group of women, because of their previous degrees, would receive an accelerated certificate to get out into the 40 United States hospitals, which were in earnest need of aides to help their wounded soldiers.

I lived in the Lewis home on 19th and Glisan Streets in Portland, Oregon; the home was a beautiful property on the corner of 20th Street. The family was lovely and kind from the moment we met. It was close to the college and I walked each morning to the campus through the woods, which was very quiet and peaceful.

From the beginning of the first courses, the new students were off like Trojans. I delighted in teaching the ladies and was inspired by their youth, adoration, and willingness to learn and help others. I taught them with my whole heart and passion about all I knew of physical therapy. I shared all that I had learned and believed. One belief I stressed was that a physical therapist should keep up with the latest in her profession so that when the latest techniques come along; she knew of them, so that she may be of the greatest service to her patients.

It was a key that these women understood that they were part of an inauguration group of a woman that was creating an innovative line of work. I often said, "Reconstruction is a new word, for a new work."

My second class began in the fall on August 8, 1918 after I received a letter from Reed College, from William T. Foster, acknowledging my hard work and value to the school. They offered me $200 a month, room and board, and expenses until the first of January 1919.

W. T. Foster, the President of Reed College, sent a telegram on August 22, pleading the case as to how important it would be for me to stay teaching the women long-term. The first course I taught at Reed College has been credited as the first school of Physical Therapy in the United States. After training hundreds of women to become reconstructive aides at Reed College, the Surgeon General needed me to pack up and travel to other cities to train more teachers and students, who would go on to help take care of the overwhelming number of wounded soldiers. I taught at Reed College until the end of 1919.

Before I returned home to Boston from Oregon, I requested a leave of absence for a couple of months before starting work again. On January 1, 1919, I received a letter from the War Department.

Since I was already on the West Coast, I decided to grant my love of travel and plan an itinerary worth writing about. Since I was already on the West Coast, I decided to grant my love of travel and plan an itinerary worth writing about.

78

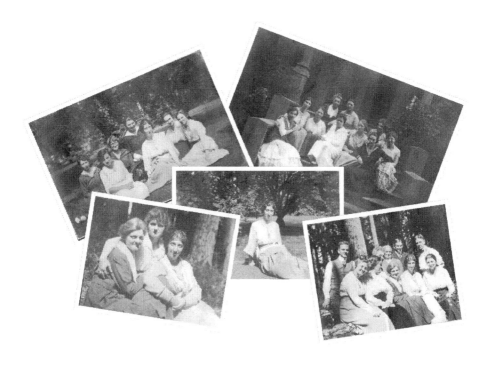

Mary and students at Reed College grounds in Portland, Oregon.
Mary in center photo among others.

I took cable cars with a shrill of delight and was awestruck by the tremendous view of the bay and the Golden Gate windmills. The enchanting city had been resurrected after it's devastating earthquake, fires, plague and political corruption in the early 1900's. The new buildings and city hall were lead by Mayor James Rolph. His leadership helped to assist in the citizen's reversal of fortunes.

I must come back to someday. Then I headed south to Los Angeles and walked on the Santa Monica Beach, where the sun was so warm and I observed people amassed in tented camps along the beaches. The warm weather took me further southeast to Palm

79

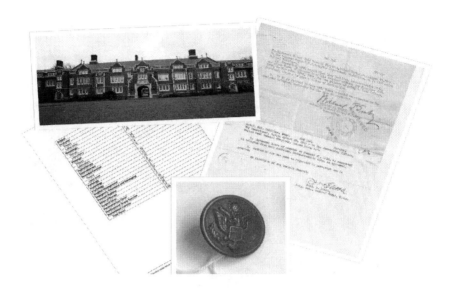

Reed College main building, PT curriculum feom 1919 and Mary's on leave of absence

Springs to see the pure white sands of the desert sprinkled with palm trees. My last stop was the great Grand Canyon, where the deep carves of the desert red rock made a canyon and river so wild that only the bravest of hearts could attempt to conquer the Colorado river blazing the trail at the bottom of the gorge.

In February 1919, I traveled to Pittsburgh on temporary order to organize and establish another physical therapy department at the United States General Hospital No. 24. It was hard work, but I was always up for a new challenge. After four weeks of uphill struggle, I decided to take a few weeks off for a much needed vacation.

When I returned from my vacation, I received a letter on March 12, 1919 from the War Department Office of the Surgeon General J. L. Hiller asking me to report for temporary duty and that I was to go immediately to Walter Reed Hospital on the 14th.

On May 18, I received a letter from War Department Office of the Surgeon General, from Carl R. Darnell, who approved an order for me to be reappointed as a Reconstruction Aide in the Medical Department of the Army at $50 a month prescribed by Section 1757.

I attended the Congress of American Physicians and Surgeons in June 1919 in Atlantic City and was inspired to hear Dr. Harvey Cushing speak. He said, "This has come to the minds of all, this new profession for women is as important as the nursing profession, and may arise through their invaluable services of the reconstruction aides."

On August 22, L. T. Howard ordered me in the Surgeon General's office to travel to other army hospitals to train their new students. I went to Fort McHenry, Maryland besides Fox Hills; Williamsbridge and Plattsburgh, New York; and Stanford. Then to San Francisco to see more applicants and teach the teachers a few classes, and visited the University of California to write out an emergency course for them to give their Department of Education. Afterwards, I traveled to Pittsburgh to help set up another physical therapy department.

However, because of World War I, there were many injured soldiers, injuries that caused the physical therapy profession to grow, and they named the new industry "rehabilitation therapy." In the United States alone there were over four million mobilized forces and 116,708 killed soldiers, 204,000 wounded soldiers, and 4,500 prisoners of war or missing soldiers.

In America, there were over 200,000 United States wounded soldiers coming home from World War I, but what would happen to them after their initial care? Before the end of the war, the schools and colleges had trained almost 2,000 women, about 300 of who served overseas.

The United States Surgeon General wrote afterwards, "These young women furnished the medical department by their intuition and have been selected with the greatest care, not only from the physical and education standpoint, but also from that of personality. The thorough training these aides received at Reed.

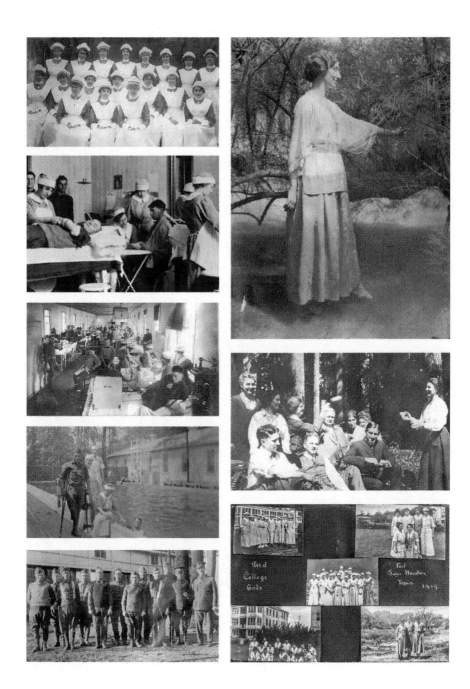

Mary teaching women at Reed College, injured soldiers' quarters, Mary with others enjoying time in the wilderness, and groups of women Mary trained.

College has made them valuable aides in the treatment of the sick and wounded soldiers."

During this time, I refined my physical therapy curriculum for my book, in addition to documenting more of the history of physical therapy. By 1919, 45 hospitals throughout the country had physiotherapy facilities and employed over seven hundred reconstruction aides. There were now over 50,000 war veterans, of which half of those were disabled during their active duty, and were being treated at these facilities. Treatments concentrated on calisthenics, including corrective exercises, passive exercises, sports and games, massage, hydrotherapeutic modalities, with assistive and adaptive equipment.

They promoted me to the Superintendent of Reconstruction aides on October 14, 1919 ordered by the Commanding Officer, Frank B. Granger, the Major of the War Department Office of the Surgeon General. I would later become the Head of Reconstruction Aides in the Medical Department and executed the oath of office under appointment on October 16, 1919.

I spent half my day at the hospital and the second part of the day assisting the Surgeon General's office with the management and staffing of the United States Army's Physical Therapy departments. I wrote many letters to the therapists that had been discharged and returned to civilian activities. I wanted to discover what they thought of their experiences, along with the standards and the future of our profession.

I lectured at different orthopedic surgeon's classes teaching treatment protocols that could be prescribed to post-surgical patients. I was also a professor for courses on physical therapy for reconstruction aides and received $800 to $2,000 according to the class size.

Over the years, I met many courageous veterans and could see how they responded to our treatments and change in their attitudes

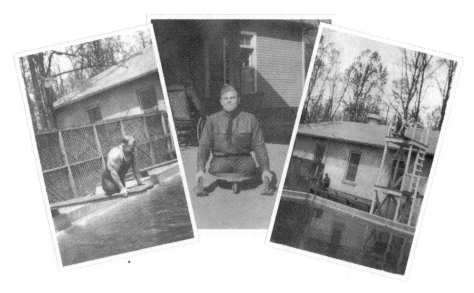

Captain Fletcher, a double amputee patient at Reed College and
World War I wounded soldier

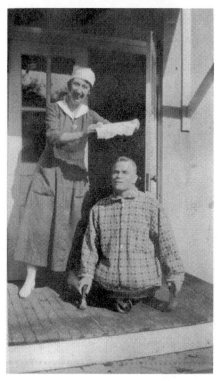

as their therapy progressed. Since there were no other options for them, some were discouraged and others cautiously optimistic as to the outcome. After all, we were the first practitioners who were paving the way for both patients and therapists in this new profession, and both starting with a clean slate of the unknown.

I remember one case; he was known around the hospital as "Fletcher" and he came home from the battlefield as a double amputee from the pelvis down. He had lost half of his body in the war, yet he survived. We worked with him for months and he slowly regained his upper body strength, recovered from his massive wounds and found his faith. He was so happy and optimistic despite no longer having any legs. He would fly around the hospital grounds on a self-made dolly rig with steel rollers underneath, pushing his upper body around as if he was a schoolboy having fun.

One day he told us he would like to take a dive into the pool to swim around. We were not sure what to think and so a group of us followed him outside to watch what he would do. We observed with amazement and satisfaction as he climbed the ladder with his long, strong arms onto the diving board, pulling himself on the ladder one-by-one. Then he used his hands to scoot out to the end of the board. He waved at all of us proudly, looked down at the water, and made a perfect dive with his arms outstretched into the pool. We all cheered for him as he rose out of the water with tears streaming down his cheeks—and he wasn't the only one.

7

A LIFELONG COMMITMENT TO TEACHING PHYSICAL THERAPY

In 1920, physicians changed reconstruction aides' designation to physical therapists. Physicians felt that these aides provided what was needed to help those wounded at war. Also, that they operated at a technician level and only under the physicians direction, that is why the name was changed.

Physical therapy methods were based solely upon the known facts of the human anatomy and physiology. The practice of these methods requires an acquaintance with the pathological conditions and symptomatology, together with knowledge of laws of electrophysics.

In February, I wanted to document some of the work and possibly write a comprehensive book on physical therapy about the work we were doing at the hospital. I sent a letter and requested permission to take any photos of the physiotherapy department and on February 6, 1920, I received a letter from Harry A. Bishop, Captain Medical Corps, the Director of Physical Therapy at Walter Reed Hospital, granting me permission.

As I continued to work for the army, I also gave lectures, continued to research, and worked on my book about physical therapy. After all of my education, attending a conference and teaching, I felt it was important to write down my thoughts and ideas on the new profession of physical therapy. I wanted to share this vital work, not only for students but also for women who have passed through

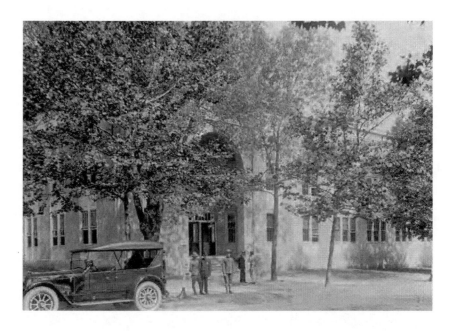

The Surgeon General's office, where Mary took over for Marguerite Sanderson to oversee the United States Army's Reconstruction Aides in Washington, DC

short intensive courses of therapy and were practicing therapists so they can reach a higher standard of efficiency.

On April 24, 1920 I received a letter from the War Department Office of the Surgeon General to increase the allowance for my work. Lieutenant Colonel Hard D. Corbusier wrote to inform me that the Mayo Clinic initiated a training program in physiotherapy on June 11, and I was to go and assist them in their endeavours.

When I returned, I realized that while I loved working for the Surgeon, it was time for me to move on. Sanderson returned to the United States and resigned because she was getting married. Shortly thereafter, Dr. Granger resigned, and at the same time, some of the emergency hospitals began to close down, so I felt it was time for me to also resign from the United States Army. It was perfect timing as Dr. Brackett had been asking if I wanted to come work for him in Boston which was a perfect job for me because I wanted some time off to visit my family and friends in England.

On June 15, I finally received a letter from the Surgeon General with my appointment form, service record, and the date of my honorable discharge from C. C. Whitcomb, Colonel of Medical Corps, who expressed his appreciation for my faithful performance of duty.

While my career in the United States Army had ended, it was written many years later that the magnificent accomplishments of the physical therapy in World War I were due in large measure by my vision and guidance. It seems funny how I simply looked on that time in the army as my destiny and profession. My enthusiasm for the work was boundless and, I hope, infectious. I only wanted to inspire and be a role model to other aides on how we could be of service to those who were suffering.

Before I left Washington, DC. I sent letters out to hundreds of physical therapy aides to inquire if they would like a national organization to be formed for them and for them to send me their ideas. There was a resounding yes. That was the first step, and a way to band together to form some type of American Physiotherapy Association.

It seemed to me this would be a great opportunity to continue our profession's work and create a national standard. A formal organization would not only recognize our newfound profession but also create a strong foundation for the future. At last, I saw the mammoth potential of this essential medical field and was determined to do all I could to bring it to the next level. We would form an organization that would change members' lives through a more cohesive and recognized profession. A vocation that I hoped would become an accepted household practice in the future. It seemed to me that once the doctors and surgeons could see the benefit and necessity of physical therapy for their patients, who

89

MASSAGE
AND THERAPEUTIC
EXERCISE

BY

MARY McMILLAN

Assistant at Sir Robert Jones' Clinic, Southern Hospital, Liverpool, England, 1911–1915; In Charge of Massage and Therapeutic Exercise at Greenbank Cripples' Home, Liverpool, England, 1911–1915; Director of Massage and Medical Gymnastics, Children's Hospital, Portland, Maine, 1916–1918; Chief Aide, Walter Reed Army Hospital, Washington, D. C., 1918; Instructor of Special War Emergency Course, and Director of Reed College Clinic for Training Reconstruction Aides in Physiotherapy, Portland, Oregon, 1919; Supervisor of Aides in Physiotherapy, Medical Corps, U. S. A., Washington, D. C., 1919–1920; Associated with Dr. E. G. Brackett, Boston, 1920–1932; Director of Physiotherapy "Courses for Graduates," Harvard Medical School, 1921–1929; Chief Physiotherapist, Peiping Union Medical College, Peiping, China, 1932.

THIRD EDITION, RESET

PHILADELPHIA AND LONDON

W. B. SAUNDERS COMPANY

1932

Massage and Therapeutic Exercise by Mary McMillan

PREFACE TO THE THIRD EDITION

SINCE the second edition of this book was published there has been a great deal of research in various pathological conditions that are treated by physiotherapeutic measures. In order to incorporate some of the more recent theories regarding lateral curvature of the spine and the later forms of treatment prescribed, the chapter on Spinal Curvature has been re-written.

Much research and clinical matter has been published of recent years regarding the etiology and the manner of classification of the different types of arthritis. That the student may be brought in touch with this important phase of physiotherapy work, the chapter on arthritis has also been re-written.

The author has tried to simplify the material in the chapter entitled "Movements of Joints".

New illustrations of exercises and revised illustrations on arthritis have been added to the text.

MARY McMILLAN.

BROOKLINE, MASS.,
July, 1932.

Preface to book, Massage and Therapeutic Exercise, by Mary McMillan

CONTENTS

PART I—MASSAGE

CHAPTER IX

CHAPTER X

CHAPTER XI

PART II—THERAPEUTIC EXERCISE

CHAPTER I

CHAPTER II

CHAPTER III

CHAPTER IV

CHAPTER V

CHAPTER VI

CHAPTER VII

CHAPTER VIII

CHAPTER IX

CHAPTER X

ing the proper attention to this early sign, it is often possible to prevent or at least postpone the development of gangrene, although there is one form in which this is impossible, but fortunately this form is comparatively rare. The author discusses the pathogenesis of intermittent claudication, giving especial attention to the disturbance of the arterial innervation. He mentions several contributing factors, such as an excessive use of condiments, overexertion, traumas, infections, exposure to cold and particularly nicotine. Observations in several hundred cases convinced him that nearly all patients are smokers and that they are highly susceptible to nicotine. He points out that intermittent claudication is often erroneously diagnosed as flatfoot neuritis, muscular rheumatism, gout, varicose veins and periostitis. The prognosis is not always as unfavorable as is often assumed, for a rational prophylaxis in the form of frequent lukewarm footbaths, proper care of the nails, suit-

able footwear, and protection against injury, overexertion, heat and cold can prevent gangrene. The author evaluates the various therapeutic measures that have been recommended for intermittent claudication. The fact that the benign form reacts to many medicaments has led to the recommendation of many preparations. Of the various forms of roentgen treatment (irradiation of the vessels, of the lower portion of the spinal column, or of the suprarenals), the first two are occasionally effective. Galvanization and short wave therapy have also been tried, but the author found the latter ineffective. He advises caution in every form of heat application, because angiospasm may result. In evaluating the much disputed sympathectomy, he points out that indiscriminate use has brought it into discredit. He considers it justifiable in cases that are refractory to other measures and in those in which gangrene threatens.

Book Reviews

LIGHT THERAPY: By Frank Hammond Krusen, M.D., Director of the Department of Physical Medicine, Temple University School of Medicine, Philadelphia. Foreword by John A. Kolmer, M.D., Dr. P. H., D. SC., LL.D., Professor of Medicine, Temple University School of Medicine. 186 pages with 33 illustrations. New York: Paul B. Hoeber, Inc., 1933. $3.50 net.

Doctor Krusen has given us a most excellent working manual on the use of light rays—both visible and invisible—in medicine. His hope that "this book will render light therapy more intelligible" has certainly been granted.

The chapters on Physics, Sources of Therapeutic Light, Need for More Accurate Selection of Therapeutic Rays and Physiology will lead particularly to a greater understanding of the application of this valuable agent.

The book is complete with technique as a whole and as applied to various diseases said to be amenable to light therapy. The bibliography is excellent as Dr. Krusen brings forward other research workers.

Again let it be made clear that this book should be a valued member of one's working library.

PHYSICAL THERAPEUTIC TECHNIC: By Frank Butler Granger, A.B., M.D., Late Physician-in-Chief, Department of Physical Therapy, Boston City Hospital; Director of Physical Therapy, United States Army; Medical Counselor, United States Veterans' Bureau. Revised by William D. McFee, M.D., Visiting Physician, Department of Physical Therapy, Boston City Hospital; Attending Specialist in Physical Therapy, United States Veterans' Bureau; Consultant in Physical Therapy, Ring Sanitorium. Second Edition, Revised. 436 pages with 135 illustrations. Philadelphia and London: W. B. Saunders Company, 1932. Cloth, $6.50 net.

In 1929 there appeared on these pages a review of the first edition of Dr. Granger's book. This second edition has been revised and brought up to date by Dr. William McFee of Boston. The main substance of the book is unchanged but Dr. McFee has added such modern references as to that of Dr. Morton Smith's faradic unit for example. In particular has been added a chapter by George B. Rice, M.D., F.A.C.S. on Physical Therapy in the Treatment of Diseases of the Ear, Nose and Throat. The book remains, we believe an established authority on physical therapy and what may be reason-

ably expected from its various agents in certain selected diseases.

MASSAGE AND THERAPEUTIC EXERCISE: By Mary McMillan, Assistant at Sir Robert Jones' Clinic, Southern Hospital, Liverpool, England, 1911-1915; in charge of Massage and Therapeutic Exercise at Greenbank Cripples' Home, Liverpool, England, 1911-1915; Director of Massage and Medical Gymnastics, Children's Hospital, Portland, Maine, 1916-1918; Chief Aide, Walter Reed Army Hospital, Washington, D. C., 1918; Director of Physiotherapy, "Courses for Graduates," Harvard Medical School, 1921-29; Chief Physiotherapist, Peiping Union Medical College, Peiping, China. Third Edition, Reset. 359 pages with 124 illustrations. Philadelphia and London: W. B. Saunders Company, 1932. Cloth, $2.75 net.

With the mass of writing on the various phases of Physical Therapy it is with pleasure that we welcome this third edition of Miss McMillan's book. It is divided into two parts—the first on Massage and the second on Exercise—and goes effectively about its business of setting forth their technique and value.

Miss McMillan takes up the five fundamental strokes of Massage, describing each with its adaptations to the different areas of the body, and covering exceedingly well their particular therapeutic value. It is an interesting commentary that immediately after the first descriptive chapter on massage there follows one on active and passive joint movements; an excursion so to speak into the realm of exercise. Again it is an interesting commentary on the close relation between themselves and to the other physical therapeutic agents that we find her most naturally mentioning diathermy or interrupted galvanic. Chapters of exceptional value deal with such conditions as Volkman's Contracture, Torticollis, Amputations, Synovitis, Low Back Conditions and Arthritis.

The first chapter of Part Two deals in brief with the history of Therapeutic Exercise. Its last sentence contains the germ of all intelligently supervised activity. "A great thing for the physiotherapist to recognize is the time when passive work should cease and exercises replace the earlier therapeutic methods."

Concisely Miss McMillan deals with the mechanics of normal—or perhaps one should say "good"—posture and posture training including visceroptosis as well as the disalignment of the skeleton. Among various other conditions benefited by judicially prescribed and supervised exercise are mentioned empyema, asthma, hernia, cardiovascular disturbances and conditions where neuromuscular coordination are lacking.

The book is clearly printed and well illustrated. Of special value is a carefully compiled index. In a brief appendix which is an answer to frequent inquiries Miss McMillan has given from her experience a list of minimum equipment for a gymnasium, an electrotherapy department and a hydrotherapy plant.

The amount of material so well presented is amazing and this small book makes an excellent reference for both student and graduate technician.

THERAPEUTIC USES OF INFRA-RED RAYS: By W. Annandale Troup, M.C., M.B., Ch.B. (St. And.) ; Author of Ultra-Violet Rays in General Practice and The Titanium Alloy Arc. Its Uses in Therapeutics; Honorary Consulting Electrotherapist to the Portman Hospital, Blanford. Honorary Physician to the Association of Retired Naval Officers, Member of the Honorary Advisory Editorial Board "The British Journal of Physical Medicine," Member of the Royal Institution. With a Foreword by Sir William Wilcox, K.C.I.E., C.B., C.M.G., M.D., F.R.C.P. Second edition revised and illustrated. London: The Actinic press, Limited. Price, 6/6 net.

Mr. Troup has brought to his public—the British medical world—the use of the infra-red rays in a general practice. He gives a brief survey of the physics, the therapeutics and the sources of the rays before he turns to the technique of their use. He compares the ultra-violet and the infra-red rays and treats upon their combination as therapeutic agents. Many case reports are quoted to show the reasonable use of this form of heat for "those minor and simple ailments which so frequently drag on (much to the annoyance of the patient) and defy other recognized forms of treatment."

DISORDERS OF SPEECH AND VOICE: By Robert West, Ph.D., Professor of Speech Pathology, University of Wisconsin. Madison, Wisconsin: Mimeographed by the College Typing Co., 1932.

A very careful study has been reported on the various causes of the disorders of speech, emphasizing that the end result is the subject for re-education only as it is considered as a part of the whole picture of the individual. The examination, testing, analysis and charting of findings are clearly described but the book brings a desire for a sequel on the approach and re-education for such a disorder.

PHYSICAL THERAPY

This concise reference text on history contains information formerly unavailable within the scope of a single volume. It discusses:
  I. Physical Therapy from Ancient Times to the Renaissance.
  II. Massage and Exercise.
  III. Water.
  IV. Electricity.
  V. Radiant Energy.

By John S. Coulter, M.D., Assistant Professor of Physical Therapy, Northwestern University Medical School, Chicago.

No. 8, Clio Medica: A Series of Primers on the History of Medicine. Published by Paul B. Hoeber, Inc. Cloth. Pp. 142, with 15 illustrations. Price $1.50.

This book may be purchased through the Business Office of

The Physiotherapy Review, 2449 S. Dearborn St., Chicago, Ill.

NORTHWESTERN UNIVERSITY MEDICAL SCHOOL
CHICAGO, ILLINOIS
PHYSICAL THERAPY COURSE

This course, designed for Graduates of Physical Education and Graduate Nurses, will be given at the Northwestern University Medical School and in affiliated hospitals from October 2, 1933, to June 30, 1934.

Credit toward a degree will be granted for this course in the School of Education of Northwestern University.

Special emphasis will be placed on Physiology, Pathology and Anatomy, in which there will be lectures, dissection and quizzes. Special instruction and many hours of practical work will be given in Massage, Muscle Training and Corrective Exercise, especially in the treatment of the various forms of paralysis, spinal curvatures, faulty postures, fractures and industrial injuries. Instruction and practical work will also be given in Electrotherapy, Natural and Artificial Radiation, Hydrotherapy, Occupational Therapy, Physical Therapy Department Administration, and Administration of work for the handicapped.

The course will be under the direction of John S. Coulter, M. D., Assistant Professor of Physical Therapy, and Miss Gertrude Beard, R. N.

Application should be made to the

Dean of Northwestern University Medical School, 303 East Chicago Avenue, Chicago, Illinois

WAR DEPARTMENT
OFFICE OF THE SURGEON GENERAL
WASHINGTON

August 20, 1919.

Oct 6 1919

ORDERS:

      Mary McMillan, Head Reconstruction Aide in Physio Therapy, Medical Department at Large, now on duty at Walter Reed General Hospital, Takoma Park, D.C., is directed to perform the following travel, for temporary duty connected with the Medical Department of the Army:

Walter Reed G.H., Takoma Park, D.C., to U.S.A.G.H. # 2, Ft. McHenry, Md.
U.S.A.G.H. # 2, Ft. McHenry, Md. to U.S.A.G.H. # 1, Williams Bridge, N.Y.
U.S.A.G.H. # 1, Williams Bridge, N.Y. to U.S.A.G.H. # 41, Fox Hills, S.I.,N.Y.
U.S.A.G.H. # 41, Fox Hills, S.I., N.Y. to U.S.A.G.H. # 30, Plattsburg Bks.,N.Y.

      Upon completion of the temporary duties prescribed, she will return to her proper station, Walter Reed General Hospital, Takoma Park, D.C.

      A delay of twenty days, accrued leave with pay, is authorized before returning to her proper station, Walter Reed General Hospital, Takoma Park, D.C.

      This employee is entitled to transportation and traveling expenses under A.R. 752 and 753, as amended. She will be allowed flat per diems in lieu of subsistence, in accordance with the provisions thereof, at the rate of $4.00 per day while traveling, and for the first thirty days of duty at each of the temporary stations designated, and at the rate of $1.50 a day after the first thirty days at each of the said temporary stations.

      The travel directed is necessary in the military service.

      By authority of the Secretary of War:

               M.W. Ireland,
               Surgeon General, U.S.Army

           By: *Frank B Granger*
              Frank B. Granger,
              Major Medical Corps.

Transportation from WASHINGTON, D C

to VARIOUS & Return

Issued the within name persons .... was

(ONE) on this order.

W2763637 Washington To Baltimore, Md
W2763638 Balto To New York
W2763639 "
W2763640 New York To Plattsburg ..Pullman Lower Or Seat
W2763641 " ..Pull Lower Or Seat
Q2763642 Plattsburg To New York
W2763643 " ..Lower Berth
W2763644 New York To Washington ..Lower Berth.OBSEAT
W2763645 " ..Lower Berth Or
SEAT

FSG-MES

WAR DEPARTMENT
OFFICE OF THE SURGEON GENERAL
WASHINGTON

Oct. 14, 1919.

From: The Surgeon General, U.S. Army.

To: Commanding Officer, Walter Reed General Hospital,
Takoma Park, D.C.

Subject: Discharge of Reconstruction Aide.

    1.   May Mc Millan, Head Reconstruction Aide in Physio
Therapy, Medical Department at Large, will execute oath of
office under appointment as Supervisor of Reconstruction Aides
on October 16th, 1919.

    2.   You are directed to deliver to Miss Mc Millan her
letter of appointment with the proper notations thereon of
date last paid and leave taken. Final pay voucher will be
arranged by this office.

    3.   If Miss Mc Millan has not been furnished quarters and
rations at your hospital, it is requested that she be furnished
with a letter to that effect and instructed to forward same to
this office, together with her letter of appointment.

        By direction of the Surgeon General:

Frank B. Granger

Frank B.Granger,
Major, Medical Corps, U.S.A.

War Department   oot-hws-lhe
Office of the Surgeon General
Washington.

                                  January 23, 1920

From: The Surgeon General.

To: The Commanding Officer, Walter Reed General Hospital,
          Takoma Park, D.C.

Subject: Unauthorized payments of the Increase of Compensation.

1. The monthly reports of disbursements of that hospital
for October, November and December show payments of the increase
of compensation to the following named Supervisors of Reconstruction
Aides.

              1. Elsey K. Taft.
              2. Mary McMillan.
              3. Martha King.

Upon execution of an new oath of office as a Supervisor of Reconstruction Aides, a new certificate must be made to the Secretary
of War to entitle these employees to receive the increase of compensation.

2. Section 7 of the Act of March 1, 1919, provedes

          "That where an employee in the service on June
     thirtieth, nineteen hundred and eighteen, has received
     during the fiscal year nineteen hundred and nine-
     teen, or shall receive during the fiscal year nineteen
     hundred and twenty an increase of salary at a rate in
     excess of $200 per annum, or where an employee whether
     previously in the service or not, has entered the ser-
     vice since June thirtieth, nineteen hundred and eighteen,
     whether such employee has received an increase in salary
     or not, such employee shall be granted the increased
     compensation provided herein only when and upon the certi-
     fication of the person in the legislative branch or the
     head of the department or establishment employing such
     persons of the ability and qualifications personal to
     such employees as would justify such increased compen-
     sation."

3. In view of the fact that an additional certificate is
required in the cases of the above named and the further fact that
the Surgeon General does not consider it expedient to recommend
Supervisors of Reconstruction Aides for the bonus, proper deductions

will be made on the next pay roll of the amount of the unauthorized payments and the appropriation "Increase of Compensation, Military Establishment, 1920" reimbursed in the following amounts:

Elsey R. Taft	$80.00
Mary McMillan	$50.00
Martha King	$28.00

By direction of the Surgeon General:

(signed) C.C. Whitcomb,
C.C. Whitcomb,
Colonel, Medical Corps, U.S.A.

This is a true copy.

H.J. Tindall,
Major, Medical Corps, U.S.A.

WAR DEPARTMENT
OFFICE OF THE SURGEON GENERAL
WASHINGTON

March 14, 1919.

ORDERS:

    Mary McMillan, Reconstruction Aide in Physio Therapy, Medical Department at large, now on temporary duty at U.S. General Hospital No. 24, Parkview, Pa., will proceed without delay to Walter Reed General Hospital, Takoma Park, D. C., and will report to the Commanding Officer for assignment to duty.

    The travel directed is necessary in the military service.

    This employee is entitled to transportation and traveling expenses under A. R. 982 and 935, as amended. She will be allowed flat per diem in lieu of subsistence in accordance with the provisions thereof.

    By authority of the Secretary of War:

                    M. W. IRELAND,
                    Surgeon General, U. S. Army.

                    By
                    J. L. Miller,
                    Lt. Col., Medical Corps, U.S.A.

April 24, 1920.

Memorandum for Colonel Whitcomb.

1. It is recommended that the bonus be extended to the following Aides as requested by the Commanding Officer, Walter Reed General Hospital.

    Miss Mary McMillan
    Mrs. Martha Feller King
    Miss Louise Hoyle
    Miss Elsey Taft

2. These Supervisors are occupying positions requiring administrative ability and responsibility and there is no incentive other than a desire on their part to render the necessary service to attract Aides with the needed requirements to fill these positions.

                H. C. Coburn,
            Major, Medical Corps, U.S.A.

This is a true copy

Wm. J. Tindall,
Major, Medical Corps, U.S.A.

In Reply Refer To S.G.O. 201

WAR DEPARTMENT
Office of the Surgeon General
Washington

May 8,1920.

From: The Surgeon General, U.S. Army,

To: The Commanding Officer, Walter Reed U.S.Army General Hospital,
             Takoma Park, D.C.
Subject: Increase of Compensation.

1. The Secretary of War has approved the allowance of the Increase of Compensation, $240.00 per annum, provided for by the Act of March 1, 1919, to the following named persons effective May 1, 1920.

2. Notation thereof will be made on the back of such persons' appointment and payment will be made to them from May 1, 1920, at the rate of $20.00 per month.

McMillan, Mary	Supervisor, Rec. Aides.		
King, Martha F.	"	"	"
Hoyle, Louise	"	"	"
Taft, Elsey	"	"	"

By direction of the Surgeon General:

C. C. Whitcomb,
Colonel, Medical Corps, U.S.A.

This is a true copy

J. Tindall
Major, Medical Corps, U.S.A.

were recovering from illness or trauma with rehabilitation, our profession would grow by leaps and bounds. It could now be possible for the world to accept physical therapy as a valued and respected occupation.

Dozens of letters from around the country were sent to Dr. Brackett, Dr. Granger, and myself asking for postgraduate courses in physical therapy. We came up with a course at Harvard that I co-directed and would begin teaching in 1920.

The first edition of my book, *Massage and Therapeutic Exercise*, was self-published in 1920 at a small printing press, and to my surprise, because of the increasing demand for physiotherapy in all of its branches it was picked up by the W.B. Saunders Company for mass publication. They asked me to revise the text to meet a greater need for training physiotherapists, which I happily began editing.

On July 30, 1920, I applied for a new passport, as my last passport had been issued in 1915. In August, I traveled to England to visit family and friends. After a few months of rest, I returned back to New York on October 17, on the ship Carmania, to begin work again.

8

AMERICAN PHYSICAL
THERAPY ASSOCIATION

In the fall of 1920, I began working as a physiotherapist at Dr. E. G. Brackett's office. I also worked at the Boston City Hospital in electrotherapy with Dr. F. B. Granger and Dr. Resneck. I moved to 38 Webster Street in Brookline, Massachusetts, and began working on revising my book for it's re-publication.

I was thrilled when my textbook, *Massage and Therapeutic Exercise* was published in hardcover by W.B. Saunders in the fall of 1921. I was grateful that Dr. Brackett wrote the forward for it, which shared, "It has been the desire of all of us who were occupied with the physical reconstruction of the injured during the war to preserve the resources developed during this period that they may be turned to the relief of the industrial reconstruction, which problem we shall always have with us." The book sold well and several reviews were written and thankfully were very encouraging.

One day, Lieutenant Colonel Hard D. Corbusier wrote to me asking if I would be interested in helping in the formation of a professional society of physical therapists. He advertised to all the physicians and surgeons of the country the importance of treatment by physical means, to elevate and standardize the work and place it on a more substantial basis. That ignited a new hope in me, as I had already planted the seeds earlier for an organization in June 1919. I became excited again about what our profession could become and how I could be of service to help.

With the enthusiasm of Dr. Frank Granger and Miss Harold from New Jersey—who gave their support, suggestions, and helped to spread the word—we finally decided to form a national organization that would standardize physical therapy practices, which would provide professionally trained women therapists the ability to practice in general hospitals and clinics.

One response from Janet Merrill, who would be the first secretary of the association, expressed deep interest in the forming of the new group and reviewing the proposed standards of physical therapy. Janet Merrill herself was a pioneer physical therapist, having been trained in the office of Dr. Robert Lovett, MD in Boston and was one of the first physical therapists to serve in the polio epidemic. She too was a teacher and trained personnel for emergency service in the catastrophic polio epidemic in New York and reconstruction aides at base hospital numbers five near Boston. I spent a good part of each day and night working on the American Physical Therapy Association (APTA) and felt if it ever got started, I worried it might be a let down. I wrote and confided to a close friend, "I knew your poetic nature would resent a business like protocol. Think my dear, of the number of letters that my poor incompetent self has had to plan and then judge me harshly if you dare."

In the beginning, I was often working alone since Mary Anderson was busy with schoolwork. Even though I invested many hours into the formation of the association, I still had the capacity for work and devotion to my profession and was also editing my book during this period.

Then, many of our founding Women's Physical Therapeutic Association members and I often met at Keens in New York to discuss the details of the organization. We discussed how many and what kinds of branches we would form under one physical therapy organization and other establishment specifics.

Keens was a local chophouse well known since 1885, and known as one of the best restaurants in New York City. It had a masculine atmosphere but with a European charm, with a great oil portrait of George Washington.

It was ironic our women's organization chose this historic place to meet because only men were allowed to gather and eat there up until 1905. Lillie Langtry, an actress and onetime paramour of King Edward VII, sued the restaurant for refusing female entrance. She eventually won, and the restaurant put up the sign "Ladies are in luck, they can dine at Keens and that is how we became lucky to meet there."

On January 15, 1921, a group of about 30 of us—and five doctors—met for the first time at Keens Chophouse in New York City and worked together on the preliminary work needed to create this historic organization. Many of us continued to meet and spent a good part of each day and night in January discussing the Physical Therapy Association, but I still had my reservations that after all our hard work it might be a let down.

It was decided that in order to become a member of the organization, a woman had to graduate from college in physical education, with additional training and experience in massage, therapeutic exercise, and some knowledge of electrotherapy and hydrotherapy.

In the midst of our planning, we had heard a great deal about different grass roots physiotherapists groups who had been organizing local associations around the United States. We learned there were already chapters set up in Los Angeles and San Francisco, California; New Haven, Connecticut; Chicago, Illinois; Portland, Oregon; and Washington, DC. These strategic organizations joined together and we asked them for any suggestions—no matter how trivial—to help us devise a plan. It was these organizations that were key to us building what would be our future organization.

109

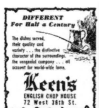

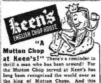

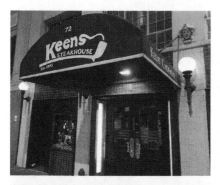

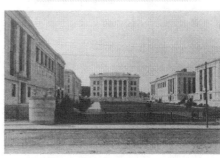

Schools and Courses, Old and New

Harvard Medical School Post Graduate Course in Physical Therapeutics

A post graduate course in the various branches of Physical
Therapeutics is being offered by the Harvard Medical School ex-
pressly for service and ex-service women. The term will extend
from July 5 to August 15 inclusive. Dr. F. B. Granger will lecture
on the theory and practice of electro-therapy. Dr. E. G. Brackett's
subject includes hip strain, back strain and their treatment by physiotherapy. Dr. F. J. Cotton will take up the curative value of physiotherapy, in pre-operative and post-operative surgery. There will be
lectures and clinical work in the theory and practice of therapeutic
exercise in cardiovascular conditions, in various types of brain and
cord lesion paralysis, scoliosis and posture training. The course
will include a review of anatomy—especially of kinesiology and of
muscle training in the after care of infantile paralysis.

Daily clinics will be held at the Massachusetts General, the
Boston City, and the Peter Bent Brigham hospitals. Theory and
practice of massage in special cases, and therapeutic exercise including hospital clinical work, will be under the direction of Miss
Mary McMillan.

Applications for enrollment should be made as soon as possible.
Tuition for the course will be $30.00, registration fee $5.00. For
further particulars write to the Assistant Dean, Harvard Medical
School, Boston, Mass.

Harvard Medical School Courses for Graduates

An eight weeks' course of instruction in physiotherapy is offered
to properly trained women by Dr. Arthur T. Legg and Dr. James
W. Sever, under the auspices of the Harvard Medical School. Instruction will include functional and sectional anatomy, diseases of
joints, scoliosis and posture training. Special attention will be
given to the treatment of infantile paralysis. Clinics will be held at
the Children's Hospital, the Harvard Infantile Paralysis Clinic, the
Massachusetts General Hospital, the Cambridge Hospital and other
allied institutions. The course will run from June 12 to August 5,
inclusive. All clinical supervision will be under the charge of Miss
Janet B. Merrill, director of the department of Physical Therapeu-

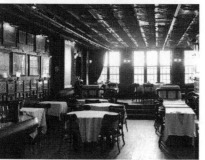

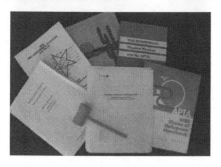

Keens restaurant in New York City where Mary and a small group of others met to create the APTA and Harvard P.T. class Mary taught for eight years

OFFICERS AND EXECUTIVE COMMITTEE
A. W. P. T. A.

President
MARY McMILLAN   38 Webster St., Brookline, Mass.

Vice Presidents
BEULA KADER   Whipple Barracks, Prescott, Ariz
EMMA HEILMAN   Phys. Ed. Dept. Reed College, Portland, Ore.

Treasurer and Secretary
JANET B. MERRILL   Children's Hospital, Longwood Ave., Boston, Mass.

Executive Committee
HAZEL FURCHGOTT   Jordan Ave., San Francisco, Cal.
MARIEN SWEZEY   Gary Hospital, Gary, Ind.

EDITORIAL STAFF

Editor-in-Chief
ELIZABETH HUNTINGTON   37 West Cedar St., Boston, Mass.

Assistant Editor and Advertising Manager
ISABEL H. NOBLE   P. H. S. 26, Greenville, S C.

Assistant Editor and Business Manager
ELIZABETH WELLS   46 Waverly St., Brookline, Mass.

News and A. E. F. Editors
INGA LOHNE   34 Emerson St., Brookline, Mass.
RUTH EARL   59 Delap St., Jamaica, L. I., N. Y.

Advertising Assistant
MATTIE HINDMAN   P. H. S. Hospital 30 Drexel Blvd., Chicago, Ill.

Subscription Manager
MARION DAWSON   669 Washington St., Brookline, Mass.

Foreign Correspondent
JOSEPHINE BELL   Station Hospital, Coblenz, Germany

P. T. Review

| VOLUME I | MARCH 1921 | NUMBER 1 |

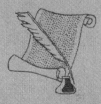

Published by
American Women's Physical
Therapeutic Association

PT Review cover for first publication in March 1921

THE "P. T. REVIEW"

Volume 1	March, 1921	Number 1

Temporary Editorial Board

Editor-in-Chief .... Isabel H. Noble
Business Manager and Assistant Editor .... Elizabeth L. Wells

The "P. T. Review"

The "P. T.Review" makes its first appearance under many difficulties.

The work has been done entirely by volunteers. We trust that our readers will be lenient about any sins of omission and commission. As the editorial work is new to us, we hope to improve as time goes on. This issue, therefore, is no criterion, as our aim is to make each copy an improvement over its predecessor.

This issue has been delayed in order that the members might be informed of the results of the election.

****

Our Aim

One of the main objects of our publication is to secure a medium through which physicians and Aides can more easily get in touch.

American Women's Physical Therapeutic Association

The necessity for a National Physical Therapeutic Association has made itself manifest throughout the country. During our period of Service, rare friendships existed. The invigorating "pull-together" feeling was so strong that those of us who are back again in civilian life feel the need of national association that will sustain these ties that should not be severed. Beyond this, standardization must be considered in order to attain the efficiency that rightfully belongs to our profession. This can only be done by united effort.

Previous to the War emergency, physical therapeutic measures were only scientifically recognized by a limited number of the medical profession, and then rarely intelligently used but by the orthopaedic surgeon.

The result of physiotherapy has no better exponent than the physically reconstructed soldier.

There seems to be a feeling by many that the requirements for entrance into the National Association as stated in the circular drawn up by the Temporary Committee were too exacting. The matter has received much consideration and the decision is strongly in favor of assuming a high standard. Each person who received a notice of the Association is eligible as a charter member.

It is feared that oversights have occurred in mailing circulars, especially among the A. E. F. Aides. Every member is urged to help rectify any errors by sending information to the secretary.

The Forming of the American Women's Physical Therapeutic Association.

This Association was started in the early part of 1920 by a Committee of the Walter Reed. At first, invitations were sent only to those who had left the Service; consequently, the Association did not gain ground very fast as there were still many Aides left. In December of last year about 800 circular letters were sent to those both in and out of the Service who, it was thought, would be interested and would want to join. The response was most enthusiastic and things moved with more speed.

Each girl who replied received a blank and was asked to nominate a president, two vice-presidents, a treasurer and two members for the executive committee. The secretary was to be appointed later by the committee. 120 Forms were returned. From these, the nomination committee compiled a ballot which was sent to approximately 200 girls, each paid-up member of the Association receiving a blank with the request that it be returned by March 24th. On that date, the nomination committee will meet and count the votes.

Upon the declaration of the ballot, our Association will be properly launched and it will be up to us to see that it is kept not only floating, but gathering more and more speed from our united efforts towards furthering its aims.

Officers and Executive Committee Elected for 1921

The vote for officers and members-at-large of the executive committee for the ensuing year has resulted in the election of the following members: President, Miss Mary McMillan; Vice-Presidents, Miss Beulah Rader, Miss Emma Heilman; Treasurer, Miss Janet B. Merrill; Executive Committee, Miss Hazel Furchgott, Miss Marion Swezey.

In accordance with the Constitution the secretaru will be appointed by the Executive Committee as early as an expression of their choice can be obtained. During the interim the President has appointed Miss Janet B. Merrill, Children's Hospital, Boston, Mass., to whom all communications should be addressed.

Message From Miss McMillan

It is with pleasure and gratitude that I acknowledge the honor conferred upon me by the members of the American "Women' s Physical Therapeutic Association in my election as President. I can only say that as far as lies within me I shall do everything in my power during my term of office to live up to the trust and confidence bestowed upon me.

There is no cause dearer to my heart. There is no group of women for whom I have more affection than my friends and fellow workers of the War Department. We went through both joys and sorrows together. The difficulties of the first days are more than compensated for by the later goodwill, which our Physiotherapy Department was fortunate enough to meet with from every hospital service with which it was identified. Never before have I seen a finer spirit among a group of women. It is to foster this spirit and to help to carry it into our profession in civilian life that our Association exists.

Although we are scattered, the separation only serves to bind us closer together. That has been proved by the warmth of expression in the replies returned in answer to a circular asking for members. That circular was distributed by the temporary Committee some months ago.

The idea of a National P. T. Ass'n. is not new, but dates back to the early part of 1919. At that time about eight hundred women were still in the service-almost the full quota of P. T. Aides. The temporary committee, which was formed in 1919, sent out a number of circulars announcing the intention of forming a National Association. Many enthusiastic responses expressed great pleasure at such a project. The time was not, however, ripe for action until 1920, when aides were rapidly leaving the service. Practically all the emergency hospitals were either closed or were about to close. Then came letter s from East and West asking for information of a rumored National P. T. Association. In November of last year the temporary committee had a meeting and decided to put the Association on its feet. The results speak for themselves. At the present time there are between three and four hundred active members; inquiries and new names are coming in constantly. If we are to progress, we must have members. The Executive Committee has appointed a Membership Committee consisting of ten or twelve members from different parts of the country.

I should like to take this opportunity to express my personal pleasure at finding myself surrounded by such a fine body of enthusiastic officers. With such an Executive Committee working for the well being of our Association, we should forge ahead.

Our Executive Committee is a representative one, two members hailing from the West Coast, two from the Middle West, and two from the East Coast.

It is with regret that the Executive Committee announces that the proposed A. W. P. T. Association Convention is postponed. A consensus of opinion was strongly in favor of holding a Convention this June, at the same time as the American Medical Association. Opinions agreed that the time was too limited to make the necessary plans for such a convention and to give the members sufficient time to make plans for the summer. Since our first Convention must be a big success, it seemed wiser to the Executive Committee to post-pone it for a year. There are several reasons for trying to arrange a P. T. Convention at the same time as the American Medical Association: First, it is easier for the committee to procure a greater variety of prominent speakers; secondly, we should be lining up our Association with the A. M.A.; lastly, we hope to get reduced railway rates. We have one whole year before the next A. M.A. Convention. Why not start now to work up enthusiasm and to make our summer plans for 1922 revolve round our National Association Convention? In that way we shall make our first convention worthy of our profession and of our Association.

You will agree that we have a live wire on our Executive Committee. The San Francisco Association is the first group to become a section of the State Medical Association. Isn't that splendid news? Did we ever dream in our most elated moments that Physiotherapy would receive such recognition from the medical profession in the first year of the existence of our National Association? This movement is due to a great extent to the work and efforts of Miss Hazel Furchgott, who is the President of the San Francisco Association. Hurrah for California! We congratulate you and trust that some clay all the local Associations may follow your example.

It seems impossible for me to close this intimate talk with you, my dear friends, without holding up the ideals that as a National Association we should have ever before us.

There are eight or nine local associations; with from ten to forty members in each In addition, there is in our National Association a considerable percentage of members at large who live in small cities or towns. It is the duty of our National Association to see that the stronger groups assist the weaker, and the isolated members who have not the same advantages as members who are living in the large cities. This may be done in a thoroughly practical way if the presidents or secretaries of the local Associations will pass along to the Editor-in-chief of our "P. T. Review" a detailed account of lectures, conferences or anything else that will be either of professional interest or of educational value to the members.

It is a great satisfaction to find that the Editorial Board has already appointed news editors in various parts of the country, as well as one in Coblenz, Germany. We should have the benefit of articles that will be instructive, interesting and entertaining.

Another duty of the National Association is to keep in touch with schools and colleges that are giving courses or postgraduate courses in Physiotherapy, so as to encourage the interest of our members in further study.

One of the most important tasks of all for our National Association is to set a standard for Physiotherapy and neither in act, word, or deed to lower that standard. Before that can be attained the Association has many bridges to cross. Every year new problem s will arise that will need the help and support of each individual member, if our National Association is to mean to our profession what the "Chartered Society of Trained Masseuses" has meant for the establishment of Physiotherapy in England. The Chartered Society's certificate is becoming harder to attain every year. The holders of these certificates have a recognized standing as "professional" women. The subjects included in the Society's requirements are: Massage, Theory and Practice; Swedish Remedial Exercises, Theory and Practice; Electrotherapy, Theory and Practice. Every member must satisfy the Board of Examine of the Chartered Society that she has had a sound practical training in all these subjects before l:egistration for the full certificate is accepted . In order to obtain the full certificate, a written, an oral, and a practical examination in each subject are required.

The problems of our National Association may be different from those encountered by the London Society, but they will be quite as real. We shall require the same kind of wise councillors, and women with broad outlook and vision, at its head, along with an advisory body of medical men and women.

My hearty thanks are due to Miss Irma Harrison, who kindly acted as co-treasurer from 1920 until the election of our National treasurer. In conclusion I want to express my gratitude to Dr. F. B. Granger for his kindness in making it possible to organize our Association by allowing the work of organization to be carried on in his office.

Now that we are truly a National Association, it is up to you and to me to see to it that our foundation is laid on sound principles that will endure.

MARY McMILLAN.

Physiotherapy in Relation to Industrial Accidents

(Part I.)

By Dr. E. G. BRACKETT

There were, perhaps, no features of medical treatment connected with medicine and surgery, which, in the early years, needed more elucidation and determination of definite principles of therapy than the different forms of physiotherapy. Their value has never been questioned, but their application in these early periods certainly left much to be desired. During the later years, much time and thought have been put into this subject by those who possessed both interest and the medical knowledge and experience, with the result of an increased practical value of the methods included in this form of treatment. Perhaps no department received a greater impetus during the war than that of physiotherapy. Its value was demonstrated, its application simplified and clarified, and its importance recognized by those who previously had not given to it sufficient recognition. Its principles of application are continually being worked out and it is now being placed on a scientific footing. A Journal such as THE "P. T" REVIEW is to be welcomed to serve as a member.

These strategic organizations joined together and helped to build the American Women's Physical Therapeutics Association. There were around 270-plus members from 32 states who signed up in the first year.

On March 1, 1921, we sent out our first issue of the association's official publication named the *PT Review*. The ballot to nominate the board of directors was enclosed in the publication and to my surprise, after they counted the mail-in votes a few days later, they elected me the first President of the AWPTA.

The let down that I expected did not materialize. My first message to the therapeutic members of the association was written as its first president and was published in the June 1921 *PT Review*. In this inaugural president's message, I welcomed our new members and outlined the functions of the new association and shared that there was no cause dearer to my heart than the association.

I wrote, "The easy path in the lowland has nothing grand or new, but a total of sum of us sent leads to a glorious view." Just a year later, the association adopted its first "Code of Ethics and Discipline."

In my first presidential address I gave at our first official meeting I shared, "The easy path in the lowland has nothing of grand or new; but a toilsome ascent leads on to a glorious view." I believed if we wanted to grow and become better at our profession we needed to continue to study, evolve, and raise the level of standards so we would forge ahead more united and stronger. In that first speech I shared, "Many of us have met in various places, it makes no difference where. We are now invited to be instrumental in formulating a standard and then to assist in maintaining such a standard."

In the early days of the organization I often said, "Early members of the first convention did not join and say what can I get out of it, they said I intend to join to see what I can make of

120

my profession and to see what I can do to create and maintain standards." How well they succeeded is a matter of history. The dedication and leadership of the charter members were to guide their association successfully through many more years.

In August 1921, physical therapy hit the scene of politics. The Democratic Party's Vice Presidential candidate, Franklin Delano Roosevelt, was taken by a severe case of poliomyelitis. He could not walk and it was difficult to do everyday tasks like eat, write, or walk. FDR was informed about the great strides in physical therapy and about the healing waters at the Meriwether Inn in Warm Springs, Georgia. They offered a physical therapy program in addition to the healing springs that was reported to cure paralysis. He went there and began to swim in the waters and soon he was relieved of his paralysis. After that, FDR spent a great deal of time in Warm Springs.

In 1922, the association changed its name to the American Physiotherapy Association (APA) and men were also admitted, and in the mid-1920s, the American College of Physical Therapy later became known as the American Congress of Physical Therapy.

In addition to the war veterans and the poliomyelitis epidemic raging throughout the country in the 1920s and 1930s, these conditions helped to increase the need for more trained physical therapists. During World War II, radical medical improvements happened because of the trial and error of so many surgical techniques on patients. These advances led to mounting numbers of survivors with many disabilities they did not know how to cope with.

Beginning in 1924, Mary Merran and I taught two of the first post-World War training courses at Harvard Medical School, where Dr. Frank B. Granger was the Co-Director of the Physiotherapy postgraduate courses 441 and 442. We were each paid $3,200 to

121

$3,700, which varied by class size and was a great deal of money back then.

On June 18, 1924, I applied and was issued a new United States passport, 445230. After many years of hard work and efforts, I needed to take off some time to visit relatives and friends aboard. I also wanted to travel to other countries to see how physical therapy was progressing.

In 1927, I traveled to England on the Arabic. I then went by train to Switzerland and spent three months at Dr. Rollier's Clinic in Laysin, Switzerland, studying methods of "sun cure." Dr. Rollier's sun cure for tuberculosis for undernourished children was becoming a recognized part of modern treatment for these conditions. This was especially important to me on a personal basis, as this was the disease both my mother and sister, Lillie, succumbed to so many years ago when I was a small child.

Dr. Auguste Rollier and his colleague, Dr. Rosselet, in their clinic at Leysin—located on one of the Alps near Lake Geneva, Switzerland—had brought it to its highest perfection. During the last twenty years, over 2,000 cases of surgical bone and joint tuberculosis were treated there, and 80 percent discharged as cured. The children were gradually exposed to the sun's rays until the whole body could be healed in winter where they spent the whole day in the sun.

On September 2, 1928, I took another trip to England to spend time with friends and do more research. I sailed on September 22, 1928, and returned November 19, 1928 on Ship-America to Boston.

Many health epidemics were happening at the same time as the Great Depression. Each year, people from around the world became worse and worse off. Financial stress added to the hardship of the human condition after the war and added to the financial collapse, the crisis became more than most people could cope with.

122

My brother, Archibald McMillan, was in securities at 60 State Street in Boston and was a banker. Thankfully, I was blessed that he managed my financial estate and paychecks. He was a stockbroker and invested both my father and aunt's inheritance and built a small fortune in stocks. Lucky for me, he foresaw the Great Depression before the market collapsed and got all my stocks, inheritances, money, and funds out just in time.

In the 1930s, APA introduced its first "Code of Ethics" and membership grew to just under 1,000 therapists. Between 1930 and 1940 the United States saw an increase in both the incidences and magnitude of poliomyelitis outbreaks.

Between May and November 1934, the doctors treated approximately 2,500 cases of poliomyelitis, almost 50 new cases at the Los Angeles County General Hospital alone.

Physical therapy treatment continued to be centered on the use of exercises, massage, hydrotherapeutic modalities, heat and light modalities, and assistive and adaptive equipment.

Home care was desperately needed and evolved during this time. Physical therapists became "on call" and provided their skills in rural homes, adapted equipment for patients, and provided braces and splints.

The Association required members to have graduated from an approved school of nursing, passed approved courses in physical therapy in a physical education and nursing graduate program, and have completed one year of practice within two years of graduation. In 1938, the March of Dimes created a coin collection and the National Foundation inaugurated it for infantile paralysis and distributed funds at the local level for various programs related to poliomyelitis. This group was founded by President Franklin D. Roosevelt on January 3, 1938 as a response to the United States epidemic of polio, a condition that can leave people with permanent physical disabilities.

Besides the treatment of poliomyelitis, in the late 1930s, physical therapy practice continued and was dominated by the treatment of wounded World War II veterans. During this time, federal legislation recognized women physiotherapists as members of the Army Medical Department, which before that time had only recognized men.

The first Social Security Act, which later had a major impact on the provision of physical therapy services to the elderly in the United States, was passed by Congress in 1935 and initiated the old-age retirement system, which employees and employers financed through payroll taxes.

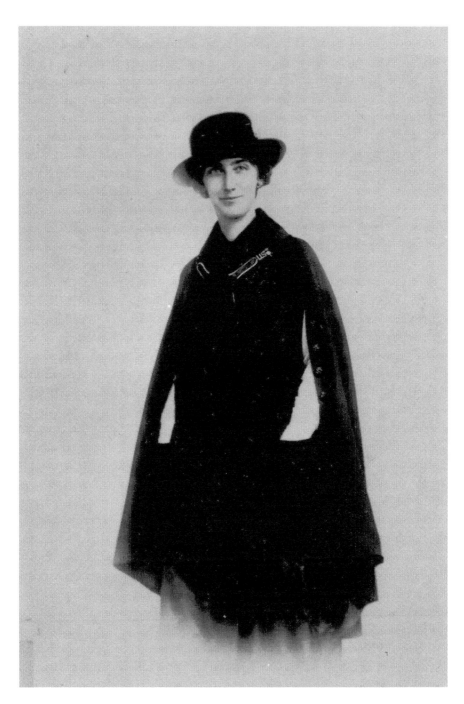

Mary McMillan in United States Army uniform

The War Isn't Over Yet for These Fox Hills Cripples

Wounded Soldiers at the Big Staten Island Hospital Say Season Isn't "Closed"

By Wilbur Forrest

A THOUSAND wounded soldiers still under treatment at the Fox Hills Hospital on Staten Island feel that New York has called for forgotten their relatives.

WOUNDED soldiers at the Fox Hills Hospital resting "in French" in leisure laboratories in their study of French

FOREIGN-BORN soldiers at Fox Hills spending their convalescent studious English

AN exhibition and sale of handwork by disabled soldiers at Fox Hills

THE days are numbered out at the Fox Hills Hospital's hobby rooms

A WOUNDED soldier at Fox Hills practising the use of his new crutches

German Society Has Nothing Left to Look Up To

By William C. Dreher

THE NEW YORK HERALD, SUNDAY, NOVEMBER 12, 1922.

5

Stepdaughters of the Army

By AN ARMY RECONSTRUCTION AIDE.

YESTERDAY we were four years distant from the signing of the Armistice. The day found us looking at the case of the disabled ex-service man with a casual aloofness. When he got back into civies, he failed to provide us with thrills. He is costing us a great deal of money. We have been told that he is lazy, unappreciative and improvident. He has even got drunk, thieved and murdered. Yes. But, as he used to say with his delightful swagger, "I'll tell the world," when the stage was set, he played the hero well. This is not a story of how he went over the top but of how he faced his shattering experience—deafness, blindness, paralysis, loss of limb and limb, disfigurement to the degree of repulsiveness —while he was in the hospital.

In 1917, like every other woman in the country, I was simply aching to get into the service. Possessing none of the qualifications for scrubbing hospital floors, for driving ambulances in France, for making pies back of the firing line, I, a school

the more complicated of the neuro-surgical and the uro-plastics, those men for whom the knife or other artificial agencies were to create noses, ears, jaws or chins.

They usually arrived at night with no waving of flags or playing of bands. I shall never forget the first large group I saw waiting to be assigned to quarters. There were about a hundred of them. The ambulatory patients sat on their kit bags, the others lay on stretchers, placed temporarily on the floor. The lights seemed very dim, the white, worn faces stood out in sharp relief against the shadows. All were uncomplaining all a little dazed looking; all silent. It was not of such a homecoming as this that they had dreamed when they waited for dawn in the trenches.

By the middle of September the hospital was functioning like a ninety horse power car. All day long fumes of ether came from the operating rooms where forty-thousand-a-year surgeons toiled on the pay of majors and captains. A full quota of

flapper, the girl of the twenties, the woman of the thirties, the forties and even of the fifties. She was the patriotic enthusiast who had taken a six weeks' course somewhere; she was the highly trained professional worker. Occasionally she was the girl who frankly wanted to get married; now and then she was the poseur who longed to be a ministering angel. In the main she was the capable, energetic, American girl who desired to do her bit. At her best she was a sort of liaison officer between the disabled man and life.

It transpired that through the very nature of her service and of her official status she had greater opportunities than either the doctor or the nurse to come close to the souls of the men. As for her status she was merely the stepdaughter of the army. Uniformed in blue and white in the hospitals and in dark gray and maroon on the street, she might wear the button, but not the insignia. Such privileges as insurance and one cent a mile

him, "if they had knocked all my teeth out I believe that you would be willing to chew for me."

When one happened to show the aching wound for a second he always managed to cover it up with a gallant gesture. There was the blind Captain, a surgeon of 45, who interrupted my reading one night with an allusion to his home. I asked if he were married and saw instantly a tightening of the clenched fingers, an involuntary scowl. "Thank God, no," he said in a vehement tone. Then, "Pardon me. Please read on. Make it—let's see—The Handmaid of Elymen!'"

There was the big Dakota rancher whose teacher asked him if he ever swore. "I used to," he answered. "But what's the fun of doing it now? I can't hear myself." And there was an Irish American whom an aid surprised one day pulling his thick hair in agony. As she turned to leave, he called her back. "Want a look?" Again he clutched his pompadour. "Indoor sports for invalided soldiers!"

That first Christmas back home we

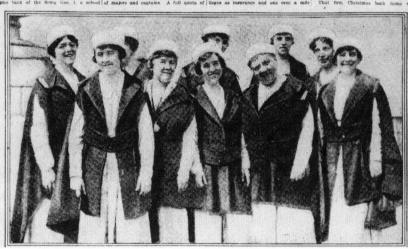

PART THREE
1932-1933

9

ROCKEFELLER TRUST
APPOINTMENT

In 1932, I made a nice little home for myself at 199 St. Paul Street in Brookline, Massachusetts.

It was a rented one-bedroom apartment brownstone near the corner of Coolidge Street. I still worked part-time in Dr. Brackett's office on 166 Newbury Street in Boston and taught at Harvard University.

I learned through Miss Eisenbrey, the Director of the Appointment Bureau of the American Physiotherapy Associations, that the Rockefeller Foundation was looking for a physical therapy professor to move to Peiping, China, to teach at the university there. I thought it would be a nice job for someone, but did not for a minute consider the possibility for myself.

I wrote a recommendation letter for another physical therapist and when I gave it to her, she asked me to find out more about the job. I discovered that it was a teaching job at the Peiping Union Medical College (PUMC). The hospital was funded and built in 1915 by the Rockefeller Foundation. They meant it to be a flagship medical institution, based on the model of Johns Hopkins University. The university focused on education, research, and practiced medicine. It opened in 1921 with the goal to train doctors and nurses as the core of China's medical profession.

My next day at work, I mentioned the recommendation I had written with Dr. Brackett and he suggested I go instead. I was stunned when he picked up the phone and immediately set up a meeting for me in New York with the Rockefeller Personnel Chief. As I pondered it, I thought, why not me? I had always been interested in seeing how other people in different parts of the world live. In my younger years and after college graduation, I went several times to visit Holland, Belgium, France, Germany, Italy, Egypt, the Holy Land, and Switzerland, so why not China?

On March 3, 1932, Dr. E. G. Brackett, MD wrote me a kind recommendation letter to Miss Eggleston at the Rockefeller Foundation to recommend me for the teaching position at the Peiping Union Medical College.

I was grateful that he mentioned that he worked at the same hospital in 1922 and highly endorsed me for my character and ability for the position. He highlighted that I was a good therapist and fine teacher, that I had a gift for putting more into the craft of physiotherapy than most, and that the Rockefeller Foundation board would be particularly fortunate if they hired me. Dr. Van Gorder, his partner, also wrote me a nice letter of recommendation. I called Miss Eggleston at the Rockefeller Foundation on March 5th to let her know how excited I was and very interested in the potential teaching position in Peiping. I mentioned how I loved to travel and appreciated the Orient and its culture. I shared that, from what Dr. Brackett told me about his experiences there, I would be very eager to go and grateful for the opportunity to interview. She told me she had already received several recommended letters praising my work and I felt somewhat embarrassed by the adoration.

My interview went well and I felt confident I was a good and experienced candidate.

While I believed they liked me very much and thought me more than qualified for the position, I heard that Mr. Green and Dr. Dieuside felt I might be too old, estimating I was over 50 years old, and it may be a big change for me. They were also concerned that I primarily specialized in orthopedic work and had done little with other types of physiotherapy, which clearly they were mistaken about.

I was told they preferred the much younger Miss Boxeth at the Presbyterian Hospital or Miss Marjorie Bennington from England, but despite my age and what they believed were my qualifications, I applied anyway. On Saturday, March 22, I filled out the comprehensive four-page Peiping Union Medical College personal history record and sent it in along with a thoughtful letter pleading my case.

It must have been a mighty miracle of God to make the appointment happen, because on June 29, Peiping Union Medical Hospital sent me an offer letter and outline of my contract terms to become their Acting Director and Chief Physiotherapist. I was shocked and thrilled to learn that the Rockefeller Committee unanimously and highly recommended my appointment for four years beginning on July 15, 1932 and ending on June 30, 1936. I was happy about the offer, and accepted the terms immediately. I believed this next phase of my physical therapy journey was to be one of the most interesting phases of my work.

THE PEKING UNION MEDICAL COLLEGE
61 Broadway, New York
PERSONAL HISTORY RECORD

Date *March 22*

Name in full _Mary McMillan._ Sex _Female._

Present address _199 St Paul St Brookline Mass._ (Until)
(Street and number) (City) (State)

Permanent address _same as above_
(Street and number) (City) (State)

Place of birth _Hyde Park._ Date of birth _25 Nov. 1880_ Race _Scottish_

Citizenship _American_ Nationality _American_ Religion _Congregationa_

~~Single, married, widowed, divorced~~ ~~Wife's name~~
(Form of customary legal signature)

~~Date of marriage~~ ~~Educational or other training of wife,~~

~~Number of children~~ ~~Age and sex~~

PHYSICAL FACTORS:

Your weight in pounds _147_ Height _5_ _7_
(Feet) (Inches)

Are you in perfect health so far as you know? _Yes_ If not, what is the impairment? _none_

Enumerate any serious sickness: Give details _never have had sicknesses except tonsilitis_
had my tonsils taken out in 1919 since that
time I have had no trouble

In what hospitals have you been a patient? When? Cause? _Tonsilectomy in the_
U S Army Hospital in Pittsburg Pa.

Life insurance: Give names of companies and dates of examinations _I have never taken out_
life Insurance

Have you ever been refused life insurance? _no_ _never applied for life Insurance_ If so, for what reason? By what companies? Date of rejection?

If either parent, or brother or sister, has died, state cause and age in each instance
Mother died after childbirth about 41 years of age
Father died of pneumonia 59 years of age

Do you use intoxicating liquors or narcotics? _I neither drink nor use narcotics of any k_

Peking Union Medical College Application for appointment

May 21, 1932

My dear Miss McMillan:

I am very happy to say that I have been authorized by
agreement of the Director, who is here, and his faculty in Peiping,
to offer you the position of chief physiotherapist in the Peiping
Union Medical College for a period of four years beginning at some
convenient date in the summer. The salary offered is at the rate of
$3000 a year payable in American currency, and traveling expenses in
going to China and in returning at the close of the appointment will
be met by the College. Salary is payable during the period necessary
for travel. Further details will be given later in the formal letter
of appointment, if, as I hope will be the case, you are prepared to
accept this.

It will be a great pleasure to the College to welcome you.

With cordial regards, I am

Sincerely yours,

Secretary

Miss Mary McMillan
199 St. Paul Street
Brookline, Massachusetts

MKE:AMP

Letter of appointment from Peiping Union Medical College

E. G. BRACKETT M.D
PATIENTS SEEN BY APPOINTMENT
TELEPHONE KENMORE 0965

WKC Mar-5 32   NKE 3/10/32   166 NEWBURY STREET
BOSTON, MASSACHUSETTS
AMP AUG-2 32 ans   March 3, 1932.

Miss Margery K. Eggleston,
    Rockefeller Foundation, China Medical Board,
        New York, N. Y.

My dear Miss Eggleston:

      Miss McMillan intends to call on you personally this week Saturday, hoping to see you in regard to the position of physiotherapist at the Peking Union Medical College. She has been approached by the American Physiotherapy Association in reference to the position.

      As I have known Miss McMillan for a number of years and am very familiar with her work, and with her as an individual, I am very glad to send you a line in regard to her capacity for this work, and since I have had personal experience with your College in 1922, I feel that I am able to speak a little more definitely than some who have not had this opportunity.

      Miss McMillan was in military service for five years during the War--three with the British and two with us, and was one of my chief workers in physiotherapy in the Orthopaedic Department. She conducted the School for the training of physiotherapists for a part of the time, and has been a teacher as well as a practical worker since the War, and has been here in my office as physiotherapist for about ten years. I can endorse her as a particularly high-grade individual, both as to character and as to ability. She is an unusually good worker, an especially good teacher, and has the capacity of putting much more into her work than that which pertains definitely to simply physiotherapy.

      I can only say that, if you should be able to obtain her services, I should consider that your Board would be particularly fortunate.

Yours very truly,
E. G. Brackett.

EGB:GM
3/9/32
ans

M. K. Eggleston
R. S. Greene
March 8, 1932

Miss Mary McMillan called on me Saturday in connection with the physiotherapy position. She has been working in Dr. Brackett's office for a good many
years and was advised by Miss Eisenbrey, the Director of the Appointment Bureau of
the American Physiotherapy Association, (who has been most patient and kind in
notifying the different branches of the Association of the position vacant in Peiping),
of our opening. She mentioned it to Dr. Brackett, and Dr. Brackett, remembering his
experiences in China, urged her not to lose this opportunity and, in fact, insisted
on her coming to New York. He and Dr. Van Gorder have both written me very nice letters
about Miss McMillan, copies of which I enclose. I also enclose copies of some letters
Miss McMillan submitted to me. Miss McMillan will fill out one of our blanks and return it to me.

The general outline of her experience is as follows: She was born in Boston,
but went to England after the death of her mother and had all of her education there.
She graduated from a school of physical education in Liverpool. Her preference was
always for the medical side and so she very soon went to London to study physiotherapy.
At one time she worked with Sir Robert Jones. During the early part of the War she
worked with Sir George Barnet. When American entered she came here. I am not quite
clear as to the order of her experience which was very varied, but she was twice at
the Walter Reed Hospital and the second time rose to be chief supervisor of physiotherapy work. She was also at Reed College in charge of the rehabillitation work there
and instruction. She knows Miss Florence Reed well and I could get information about
her from Miss Reed. She started the American Physiotherapy Association and was its
president for two years. In addition to her work in Dr. Brackett's office, she has
taught summer school at Harvard for eight years where she has been Co-Director with
Dr. Grainger. She has written a book, of which she has been good enough to say that

FORM P. 10

.r. Greene   -2-   March 9, 1932

INITIALED FILE COPY

she will send me a copy. I shall forward it to you in China.

Miss McMillan makes a very pleasant impression and I believe would be a very charming and satisfactory person in Peiping. I have two hesitations about considering her seriously. In the first place, I fear she is perhaps older than would seem advisable for an appointment to foreign work. Miss Clara Eisenbrey, you may be interested to know, is among the people who have indicated an interest. It seems to me, and I feel Dr. Dieuaide feels as I do, that the fact that she is fifty years old might make it seem better not to invite her to this new type of work. I am of the opinion that Miss McMillan is probably not far from that age, but I may be wrong. Secondly, she seems to have specialized in orthopedic work and has done relatively little of any other type. Since, however, she has been teaching physiotherapy, I should think that this consideration would be less serious.

At the moment I am most interested in Miss Boxeth at the Presbyterian Hospital, about whom, however, I have not made very many inquiries, planning to do so in personal conversation at the Medical Center. Miss Boxeth would require at least $3000. Dr. Dieuaide was pleased with the report of my conversation with her, but did not have a chance to see her. If you are not willing to pay that much, Dr. Dieuaide and I both believe that Miss Marjorie Bennington would be a very satisfactory person, say at $2200.

Miss Bennington will return to England very shortly if she does not secure any position and will probably not be available unless it is possible to make a decision shortly.

MKE:AMP
Enc.: Dr. Brackett-MKE, 3/3/32
      Dr. Van Gorder - MKE, 3/4/32
      Four letters addressed to Miss McMillan

G.in.P.

Miss McMillan   -3-   6/29/32

    The foregoing is an outline of the agreement that the College
is prepared to make with you and takes the place of a contract. The
trustees have ruled that the College cannot be bound by any understandings
other than those embodied in written communications from the Board of
Trustees, its Secretary, or the Director. If, therefore, there are any
material points relating to your appointment which have not been included
in our correspondence, kindly inform me at once, so that the official
record may be complete.

    May I have your formal written acceptance of this appointment
under the conditions outlined above?

                                        Sincerely yours,

Miss Mary McMillan
199 St. Paul Street   Secretary
Brookline, Massachusetts

MKE:LM

Enclosures
    Travel Memoranda
    Insurance and Annuity pamphlet
    Application form for Deferred Annuity

10

DISCOVERING THE ORIENT

I left Boston on July 22, 1932 and took a train to Portland, Oregon. This moment was the first step on my new adventure—a new life across the sea in China. The ride was long, hot, and dirty, and after a few short days, once I reached the city of Portland, my spirits lifted as I walked out of the train station and meandered about the quaint city. I smiled as I remembered the happy memories from thirteen years earlier when I taught at Reed College.

The good, old Benson Hotel welcomed me with open arms. Once I reached my room, it was hard to believe I only had time to wash up and, that within a few hours I'd have to start the next leg of my exciting journey. It seemed too good to be true.

My old friend from my Reed College days, Dr. Elmer Carson, came over to the hotel in his car and drove me to a most attractive house in the suburbs where we had dinner with some of my dear college and hospital friends, Dr. Otwere and Dr. Mabel. We spent the evening talking about our time shared together, helping and teaching physical therapy to others. After a lovely evening, I bid everyone a fond farewell and left for the train station. Although my train had been scheduled to leave for Seattle at 11:45 p.m., it did not come until after midnight and Elmer insisted on staying with me until it arrived.

The next couple of days I spent were in Seattle. Upon reaching the Hotel Frye, I entered the grand lobby with its reception desk, oriental rugs, upholstered seating, and ornate China vases filled with daffodils. I felt as though the décor was a wonderful foretelling of my future life in China. When I arrived in my room early in the morning, I found several envelopes and a large bunch of roses with a letter from my brother, Archie. I took a nap and when I awoke my heart warmed when I formed the roses into corsages to wear for the next few days. I kept one in a box and one to wear at my first dinner aboard the ship on Saturday.

I spent much of my day in Seattle with my poor friend Rosella who was in the hospital. Several of my old students from the college days, now living in the city, gave me a dinner party at the athletic club on Friday evening. Ruth Babb came all the way from Tacoma to join the party. I had her stay at the hotel with me the whole night. She was my old buddy, who shared a tent with me in 1919 at Walter Reed Hospital, and never shall I forget her devotion, and she was just the same sweet fine girl. Needless to say, we did not have much sleep that night and Ruth left on Saturday morning before 7:00 a.m., just a few hours before I had to leave.

Vancouver: July 30, 1932

The ship sailed from Seattle to Victoria, BC. The journey was pleasant and we reached the port around one o'clock and decided to tour the Empress Hotel. The décor was essentially English in every way—quiet and restful with lovely gardens. I breathed in the clear, crisp air as I looked out at the marina, waiting for the boat that was to take me to China.

I stood on the dock at the Esquimalt Harbor and watched the Empress of Japan glide into the port with its three amber steaming smoke stacks puffing in stride. Hundreds of men on the dock and on the water in rowboats guided and secured the boat to the dock as the crew on board scurried along the decks. The captain stepped out on a long observer deck that looked like a diving board to watch that everything was being managed just right.

The passengers gathered below the gangway and at 5:00 p.m. I followed them aboard the grand ship for the first time. It was   a clean, beautiful, and regal boat indeed.

142

A group of funny, little Chinese staff swarmed off the ship to carry our baggage. They were all dressed alike: tight fitting, black leggings from which tiny spindle, white stocking covered legs appeared. They wore long, white aprons like a frock, and black felt-heeled shoes. Truly, all I could think of when I looked at them bustling about was a swarm of bees buzzing out of a beehive.

The good ship snorted and whistled, then my heart fluttered, as I knew there was no going back to my life in America now. I discovered the Empress of Japan had a top speed of 23 knots and was known as the fastest ship on the sea.

A porter escorted me to cabin 238, opened the door, and I was surprised to see how palatial it was. The square room had light oak paneling, with trimmings and fixtures in deep cream and blue, with a poster bed to match. On my ample dressing table, I spread the handsome toilet articles the ship's greeting committee had given me, along with the kimono Kay had gifted to me, which blended in harmony with my surroundings. Never had I known a more comfy bed, which had no semblance to my old army bunk days. The room also provided an electric fan above my head in case I became too hot and an electric heater in case it was chilly.

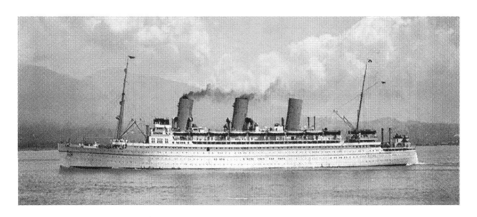

Sailing on the "Empress of Japan" 1932 to new appointment at Peking Union Medical College

The wardrobe had ample and excellently equipped storage with doors and plenty of hanging space. There were many packages, letters, magazines, and telegrams when I came into my room after dinner. Telegrams from Archie, Maud, and Kay had been delivered a couple of hours earlier than the rest of my mail and packages. I shed a silent tear when I read my family's loving words. Even though my family and I were now so far apart, I could still feel their ardent thoughts surround me and I thanked God for that feeling.

Among the pile of over twenty letters, I have a dear little note from Dr. Brackett wishing me a safe journey. In addition, I found a little telegram from a Mr. Rogers S. Greene saying, "If you are the Mary McMillan who has recently been added to the staff of the Peiping Medical Hospital, I should like to meet you early on the voyage. If you will let me know the time and place, I should be happy to call upon you." I replied that I would be in the writing room the next morning at ten o'clock and he arrived promptly the next morning.

Mr. Greene looked younger than I had expected. He was the brother of Crosby Greene, a throat specialist I had known in Boston, and also a Harvard graduate and classmate of President William Trufant Foster of Reed College. He stood tall, a slightly dark man turning bald on the crown, but otherwise no gray hairs. A quietly spoken man, keen looking, gentlemanly, about 5' 1" tall. Our first interview was pleasant and we chatted easily for an hour or more.

There was no escaping physical therapy for me on the Empress of Japan. On Sunday afternoon, I ran into Mr. Greene, who told me he had caught a cold shoulder by sitting in a draft and his head was hot to the touch. The cold was indeed in Mr. Greene's shoulder. It is known as a frozen shoulder, a condition that affects the shoulder joint, involving pain and stiffness that develops gradually, worsens, and then finally goes away. He asked my advice

144

about seeing the ship's masseur. Eventually, he agreed that I go along with him to see that the efforts of the ship's masseur were not too strenuous. I advised hot packs followed by ice packs, and then gave the shoulder a little effleurage and petrissage, kneading his shoulder expertly. He smiled with gratitude for my kind efforts to help him.

Empress of Japan: August 2, 1932

As the days passed on the ship, I found myself falling into a peaceful rhythm. The blue seas and cool crisp breezes on the Pacific calmed me as we sailed southwesterly. I spent a good amount of time in my spacious room. I would lie down with a couple of dozen rosebuds opening out each day on one side of my washboard and in another bowl of roses, sat on the opposite side windowsill, next to a vase of sweet peas and mignonettes.

I enjoyed reading my books and magazines and thought if John D. Rockefeller knew I'd have enough to keep me busy for the next few months, he might have made it a trip around the world instead of only as far as China. I appreciated it all and thoroughly enjoyed reading, writing, and having a swim on the deck besides dancing in the evening. I felt as though I was leading the life of Riley. I experienced a lazy life at sea. With strenuous days ahead of me, it was good I built up strength and rest for the future strain of work and a new culture that was unknown to me.

August 7, 1932

There were comparatively few passengers aboard; the Canadian Pacific must have been running the ship at a loss. I should think not over 50 first class passengers were aboard the ship. The menus and service were excellent and yet the dining room sparsely filled. There

145

was an especially pleasant group of British people aboard and quite a few of them going to Honolulu and then onto the Orient.

On Thursday, around ten o'clock, we steamed into the Honolulu Harbor. A beautiful morning awaited us and the thermometer registered just 79 degrees, the same temperature as the water. It seemed as if the whole island's inhabitants came to meet our ship. Hawaiian men, women, and children gathered on the shore as we eased into the landing place. Swarms of coolies in bathing trunks reeled out to greet the passengers. They seemed at home in the sea and swam like the fish.

As we drew alongside the pier, the civic band dressed in white played tune after tune of Hawaiian music—the men sang in harmony in their native anthem song of the Isles. It was a beautiful view, like nothing I had ever seen. A girl followed by a large party skipped down the brow way and they played Lohengrin's Wedding March in honor of the young bride who walked directly from the boat to the church to be married that very morning.

Everyone on shore, both men and women, wore garlands of flowers around their necks. They made leis from a variety of native flowers, among the commonly known are a large soft yellow and pink flower with a particularly powerful odor known as the plumeria. They disbursed flowers—soft pink, yellow, blue, and purple—which smelled so lovely that the whole atmosphere was delightfully fragrant.

Mr. Greene invited me along with two other ladies to drive with him around the island and have luncheon. We drove around and went to Waikiki Beach to eat at the Royal Hawaiian Hotel. We drove around the entire island of Oahu and stared in awe at the gorgeous view of the beach and coastline.

We returned to the steamer at 7:00 p.m., both excited and exhausted, and returned to my room. I discovered the captain had invited me to sit at the table. After dinner that evening, I strolled

146

to shore with him and Mr. Peaks, a Liverpolitan by birth living in Shanghai. I believe he was some type of engineer. The captain had been so kind to me and was quite an interesting man.

Oh, how I loved seeing the many interesting sites we saw by the early evening light! The captain drove us alongside a sugar plantation that went on for miles and miles, and we saw piles of sugar cane piled on trucks ready to go to the sugar press. We observed pineapple fields that were selling sweet honey pines, three for 25 cents. We noticed the pineapple factories, Libby's bananas growing up in tall trees, and one magnificent mountain range after another.

The next day, a lady passenger and I wandered ashore immediately after breakfast. We browsed around the city and viewed many unique buildings. The style chiefly of a Moorish architecture with large yards in the building's center and colorful flowers everywhere—such beauty and perfection in bloom that I had never seen before! We returned to the boat at 3:00 p.m. having spent a grand and glorious 28 hours in Honolulu.

I can remember, in my younger days, treasuring a small hibiscus plant with one or two small blossoms, whereas in Honolulu, hibiscus hedges grew in abundance. Literally miles of pink and purple flowers lined the streets. The most darling other floral specimens were the beautiful bougainvillea trees, a solid mass of deep purple flowers with shiny green leaves.

The send-off from Honolulu was even more of an affair than our arrival. For not only did a band play but also a Hawaiian singer crooned for us as paper steamers of every color were thrown in the air with joy. Almost everyone on the wharf placed garlands around the passengers' necks, of which two leis were given to me.

147

August 8, 1932

I enjoyed a warm day at sea, blue skies with the smell of tropical air. On board, the men and women dressed in white lounged on the deck, basking in the sun. Sunday evening, the captain invited a group of five passengers into his suite before dinner; a nice young American couple, Miss Moore, Mr. Green, and yours truly. They served cocktails and a very elaborate dish of hors d'oeuvres. Then afterwards, the six of us had dinner at the Captain's Table.

They compelled us to eat with chopsticks—it was my first lesson. It surprised me, but I managed to get a good deal of chow mein and rice from the bowl into my mouth with them. I had a lot of fun. On Sunday evenings they always showed a movie aboard. Two days later, we skipped a day in our lives because of the time change. Blink, it disappeared. I felt that I should never be able to reclaim this one-day entirely lost. Our week skipped from Sunday to Tuesday, not to mention turning back our watches from the twelve-thirty hour at night.

I often stood in awe on the deck looking way out in the Pacific at not a thing in sight but water. My long lazy days of relaxing were joyous. I swam each morning before breakfast and another time before dinner in the evening, either a swim in the tank or else a saltwater bath, making the most of the water of the Pacific Ocean. For the last two days, efficient Chinese boys and waiters served our luncheon on the promenade deck. It was a festive-looking scene because they had placed palm plants and shrubs on the deck with the ocean dancing in the background, which created a scene right out of a movie.

I was so attached to my Chinese steward that when I changed my table, I asked for my own dear waiter back and he kindly granted me the favor. It was quite ridiculous for the captain to have his own waiter and I have mine with just two of us at the table, yet somehow we had two stewards.

There was a very nice American lady who came on board at Honolulu. She was visiting a young niece in Peiping. I was thrilled to meet her and got to know her well. It was nice to have company for the rest of the journey. Mr. Greene told me that the college would send someone to meet me at the train station to see that I had no trouble with customs. The Rockefeller Foundation certainly was thoughtful about their employees, nothing for their comfort or well being had been omitted.

There were discussions on whether or not I should go on with the steamer to Shanghai. Mr. Greene planned to go that route and they left it to me to decide. I thought I should probably choose the direct Kobe to Tientsin route because I understood it was very hot in Shanghai at that time of year. Of course, I was interested in seeing Shanghai, but I believed I might have another chance to visit before I returned to America.

There were several boats going to Tientsin, but only two of us were to go direct to Peiping. The majority of the passengers were planning to go to Shanghai. After a busy day, I was foolish enough to fall in with the other passengers and for the large sum of two dollars hired a costume for the evening's party. It was quite a pretty one, a lady of 1830. It had a poke bonnet and white ruffled pantaloons with a costume, color effects old gold and violet. I had arranged with the headwaiter a special menu and a bottle of champagne. I also ordered a birthday cake with one large candle in the center and baked Alaska brought in flames, in honor of the captain's birthday. I asked the orchestra leader to play the "Mikado" as it was the captain's special favorite song.

I was so grateful to him, as he had been so kind to me, that this gift was a small way of expressing my gratitude.

149

I invited the lady who was traveling to Peiping besides my wonderful high chief, who also had done many nice things to make the trip more pleasant for me.

After speaking to the captain, I decided to leave the Empress of Japan after we reached Yokohama, and take an electric train trip about two hours ride to Tokyo. I planned to spend the night in Tokyo and board a train first thing in the morning at 8:30 a.m. that would reach Kyoto at 4:40 p.m. Then I planned to stay overnight in Kyoto and take an early train to Kobe and then Monday at noon, August 5, would take a small Japanese steamer to Tientsin.

I ended a most delightful trip on the Empress of Japan and Mr. Greene saw my luggage off the boat and onto the Japanese ship destined for Tientsin. I thought to myself as I left the boat, that I shall never forget my wonderful journey and dear friends I met on that enchanting trip.

August 13, 1932

Japan had much charm and wonder. When I first stepped off the Empress of Japan and placed my foot on the shore in the Orient, I felt a sense of faith in certainty mixed with fear of uncertainty. As each day passed on my journey, I learned to live by the Sermon on the Mount motto, "Sufficient unto the day is the evil thereof." And that is what I did. I did not worry about what would happen to me in the future. I took my life day by day with faith in my destiny.

My new American friend and I arrived in Yokohama safely and discovered that most of the city had been recently rebuilt due to it being destroyed on September 1, 1923 by the Great Kantō earthquake. We learned over 30,000 people lost their lives and injured another 40,000. After the earthquake, the Japanese became angry because they believed the Koreans, who lived in Kojiki- Yato slums, had used black magic to create the earthquake and a

150

rebellion broke out. I reflected on how human beings can still thrive and rebuild even after so much loss and misfortune.

We went on a brief driving tour of the city and beheld the beauty of the Yamashita Park located on the waterfront. They created it from the earthquake rubble and it had a large green lawn with flowerbeds, foundations, and memorials.

We delighted in the view of Mount Fuji in the distance from the electric train as we rode towards Tokyo. The upper part of the mountain was fairly well covered by clouds, but for the formation of the mountain, one of its chief characteristics was quite in evident. Our time in Tokyo went quickly and we only had glimpses of the city before we had to catch our train in the morning to Kyoto at 8:30 a.m.

Unfortunately, the same tragedy happened to Tokyo as it had in Yokohama. The Great Kantō earthquake, an 8.3 magnitude on the Richter scale, had destroyed 75 percent of their city. They persevered afterwards and built five to six story structures of concrete on wide streets and a new subway system. We observed a mix of men in American-styled suits with long wool coats and hats roaming the streets, walking alongside women in their traditional kimonos.

The next morning, we hurried to catch the special deluxe train, the only one in 24 hours that left for an eight-hour trip by express train and arrived at 4:30 p.m. I wish I could describe like a great writer some of my most vivid impressions of that perfectly delightful train trip, but will alas offer my best try.

It was one of the cleanest and most comfortably equipped trains I had ever been on. The observation car had settees and large comfortable swivel chairs all heavily stuffed with velvet cushions, covered with spotless, white linen. They decorated the observation car in Japanese style black and red lacquer, with touches of gold lamps on the writing desks. The train company provided an abundance of papers and postcards free for passengers and a courier stood close by to point out places of interest out the window. Through the glass at the rice fields, I saw fresh, yellow-green fields surrounded by wooded mountains everywhere. It was a romantic scene to look at the rice pickers, both men and women in the fields bending over in unison to perform their work. They wore traditional kimonos and on their heads were attired with something that looked like a straw lampshade covered with a rice cloth, or an old straw helmet made of the same material.

To my surprise, three of the ladies from the Empress of Japan appeared on the train ride down to Kyoto, so we all had a pleasant dinner party, an excellent meal, and the day on the train passed all too quickly.

We reached Kyoto late around 10:30 p.m. on August 14 and checked into our hotel. You see, by leaving the Empress at Yokohama, I gained a day in Japan and was the better for it. Kyoto was a perfectly beautiful resort with mountains thickly wooded on all sides. In fact, the resort sits up on a grand hill and commands an excellent view.

I had a comfortable room with a bath and slept like a top the first night. In the morning, the three American ladies and I hired a car with a courier at 8:30 a.m. to drive us around the city until twelve o'clock. We visited the temple parks, shrines, and buildings of local interest. He dropped us off at the train station and we said our farewells. They left for Kobe and I traveled alone on an electric train to the ancient city, Nara, which took just an hour.

When I arrived in the city of Nara, I hired a *jinrikisha* and for the first time had a human horse pull me along the bustling streets. I felt conscious and grief-stricken the whole two hours and wanted to get out to push the contraption myself. However, my coolie boy

152

seemed quite happy and took pride in his job. Especially when I stopped and let him choose a cold drink. I saw he picked out the biggest bottle on sale. He seemed humble and kind. We bought cakes to feed the deer in the parks. I quickly walked into and out of temples and shrines. The ancient and beautiful structures left me breathless. One temple of Buddha had 3,000 lanterns hanging around it. I strolled around the temples of Buddha and Shinto temples for two solid hours.

I returned to the beautiful Nara Hotel that sits like a palace atop a hill on the south edge of Nara Koen Park. I rested for an hour or so before 7:00 p.m. dinner. Afterwards, I spent the evening on the roof garden watching the talking picture *Trader Horn*, starring Harry Carrey and Edwina Booth, who played a lost child being worshiped as a white goddess by an aboriginal tribe. How funny it is that actors can portray us as irrational and senseless human beings.

I retired before 10:00 p.m. because I needed to be up early. I was not tired, but the eastern mind has no definite idea of time or appointments in other time zones, so I figured I might just as well get accustomed to the oriental clock anyway. Before I went to my room, I asked the hotel clerk at the desk who spoke English, although none too well, to call my room by 7:00 a.m. as I wanted to leave the hotel by 8:00 a.m.

At 6:45 a.m. the next morning, my phone rang, but I must confess it was the hardest thing in the world to get up, dress, have breakfast, and place my bag in the motorcar in time to catch the 8:30 a.m. train. The hotel, being fully two miles or more from the station, was worth it to stay longer to see the picturesque views—and it was much cooler on the hill, yet warm, but no warmer or uncomfortable then I had experienced in Boston.

The Oriental Hotel, Kobe, Japan: August 15, 1932

I reached Kobe at 10:00 a.m. and took a *jinrikisha* to the Oriental Hotel to pick up my trunks from the office. When I arrived, can you guess what I found? I walked to the cook's office located in the hotel lobby to pick up my ticket, which were supposedly reserved tickets for me by a cook's agent, who came on the Empress of Japan at Yokohama. Originally my purpose in the two hours I had allotted, which I planned it would take to get to Kobe, was to get my ticket, make sure that my trunks were put aboard the Japanese steamer, and send a telegram to the college to specify my approximate time of arrival in Tientsin.

To my surprise, they had sent a telegram that morning to cooks from the college. The telegram read as follows: "We advise Mary McMillan staying over until August 18 for a better ship, do not book her on an inferior one."

Did you ever know such consideration in your life? Mr. Greene had said while aboard the Empress of Japan, if the ship on the fifteenth was not a good one, which "I think you had better wait a couple days and go on a more modern one." The three ladies from the ship had their reservations on the Hikawa Maru on the eighteenth. I thought if they were game, then I should be to. However, faced with receiving that telegram, I decided I would be foolish to go on that boat and miss an opportunity to see something more of Japan.

It thrilled me because I would now have from August 13 to the afternoon of the eighteenth, which gave me almost six full days to tour Japan. I immediately walked down to the little steamer they expected me to leave on to explain to the lady that traveled with me on the Empress the reason of my change of plans. It was indeed an inferior cargo boat and I felt reassured I had made the right decision.

154

Afterwards, I returned to the Oriental Hotel and met a very nice young American couple, Mr. and Mrs. Brown, who were returning from the United States after their first five months furlough. They had a sweet little daughter who had not yet had her second birthday. Their ladies were also staying at the Oriental Hotel until they could find a house; they had put their furniture into storage when they broke up housekeeping in the spring before leaving. They had an *amah* to take care of the baby so that Mrs. Brown was free all day long. I never could have seen or done the things I had if it not been for their kindness and knowledge of the country and people.

The first night Mr. and Mrs. Brown took me to a real Japanese restaurant. It had a special small room privately engaged for us, and a hired geisha for entertainment. We ate with chopsticks and traditional food. This restaurant was the finest in Kobe and noted for a Japanese dish known as *sukiyaki*.

The restaurant was snuggled away among Japanese gardens with shrubs and short stubby trees on every side. Guests walked down a narrow unassuming lane and were surprised as they entered a beautifully lighted garden. There were over twenty separate rooms in this establishment, some large and very costly as to the decoration, with no furniture in any, except one low, centrally-placed table. They took us through the whole house except in the private rooms, which was occupied by parties such as ours.

On the step, a tiny maiden stooped down, took off our shoes, and greeted us in Japanese. In their stead, she placed straw-braided mules on our feet, which we wore through the different passages and rooms we passed through to get to our own special room, which my host had previously engaged. At the entrance of the room, we took off our straw slippers and walked in stocking feet to a small, low table in the center of the room. Mr. and Mrs. Brown, and

155

yours truly, all sat down on cross-legged upon cushions on the floor arranged around the table. Our little Japanese waitress arrived and prepared the table for our dinner.

They uncovered a small round hole in the table's center and placed a little charcoal-filled metal iron bowl, then placed a chafing dish over the hot charcoal. The little Japanese maiden stepped away and returned with a lovely Japanese lacquer tray, upon which were many small pewter-covered dishes. One of these meals contained what appeared to be slices of thinly cut steak and where gently placed in the hot dish, followed by green vegetables and onions. Once slightly cooked, she added a bit of salt, sugar, and black-looking sauce into the pot with a little water. They turned this mixture with the chopsticks for about ten minutes or so.

In the meantime, they brought each person a towel that had been wrung with hot-perfumed water. We used it to cleanse our hands before partaking of the meal. She then handed each of us a little handle cup and sake was poured from a hot pretty pottery vase shaped container. By the time another waitress presented herself and gave each of us a napkin and chopsticks, another maiden set down a small bowl with deliciously cooked rice.

I watched, then followed my hosts dive their chopsticks into the hot sukiyaki and then into the rice. This was my second experience using chopsticks; I didn't fair as well this time around as I did on board the Empress of Japan.

One waitress kept busy refilling the pot with meat and vegetables as the geisha performed her dance and sang. My hosts spoke Japanese sufficiently well to converse at ease. Our geisha then sang with the accompaniment of a three-string, little instrument, something like a guitar.

Dinner lasted a long time, quite a ceremony in all. Before we left the table, hot tea and hot towels, one for each, were carried on an exquisite lacquer tray and, dug out from hot-perfumed water, one handed to each person. Before we left, we strolled by a very

156

elaborate garden. We bowed back to at least a dozen geishas and waitresses, and put our shoes back on, which had been stored in a cupboard for evening.

Through the kindness and courtesy of Mr. and Mrs. Brown, I met a very charming Japanese lady, Mrs. Isida. She went to school in Yokohama and knew Mr. Greene. In fact, the school she attended in Yokohama belongs to Mr. Greene's sister. Never have I received more considerate kindness than from Mrs. Isida.

Early in the morning of August 16, my sweet, new Japanese friend dressed in a *kimono* and called for me at the hotel. We took a taxi out to view the school of geishas. They taught the girls to dance, sing, and to make themselves as alluring as possible in the entertainment profession. She also took me to attend a tea ceremonial, the Chinese considered a fine art. The girls attended a school that teaches nothing else but the tea ceremonial, which includes the arrangements of flowers—a different arrangement for each occasion, and every flower arrangement has its own significance.

I invited my little Japanese lady to have lunch with me. As she prefers Japanese food, I kindly asked her to choose a Japanese restaurant she most loved. They did a similar performance at the entrance and had us remove our shoes and wipe our hands and face with perfumed towels. We squatted on the floor on cushions and were served numerable dishes on small lacquer trays. They gave us chopsticks only for eating. The luncheon was of fish soup, rough fish, pickled fish, pickled seaweed, red watermelon, banana, white melon, and tea with rice. I just couldn't manage to eat the main dishes, but ate the fruit and rice.

We left the restaurant and drove for miles in a taxi to the home of a very wealthy Japanese lady whose father was known as the wealthiest man in Korea. The house was truly Japanese—sizeable yet simple in design, artistic, and most pleasing.

We walked up the steep driveway lined with a long grove of bamboo trees, which provided cool shade to the occupants. The house was square and had a large open courtyard with a garden. It stood on top of a hill overlooking the Pacific Ocean.

In every house of wealth in Japan, they keep one room, known as the Western Room, furnished with American-style chairs, tables, radios, and telephone. They only used the room for the various guests who visit from the United States.

They showed us first into the Western Room and a Japanese maid brought in some delicious ice-cold tea with lemon. Our hostess then appeared, a very young Japanese lady, Mrs. Taimaker. She entered, beautifully dressed in an elaborate kimono and handsomely embroidered *obi*. She asked if we preferred to stay in the room or if we would like to be entertained in the Japanese fashion. I chose to enjoy the traditional Japanese chamber.

The maid came in, took off our shoes, and we walked through the many halls. Simple but costly furniture decorated the halls with extremely Japanese ornamentation. We entered the most beautiful, square room that opened into the courtyard and gardens. We sat around a handsome red lacquered table on floor cushions.

Even though our hostess had lived a year in London, and had been educated abroad, she could not speak English. We talked for probably a couple of hours, exchanging views on different countries and people, very much as one might have in any Eastern home. Japanese food was served ceremonial style and afterwards we were offered fruit compote, cake, mixed sweets, and wine.

We walked through the gardens and they presented each of us with a bunch of carnations artistically arranged by one of their gardeners. Mrs. Taimaker walked all the way down the

158

hill with us and sent us off safely in a taxi she had ordered. I was so inspired by her beautiful gardens, I hoped to have one of my own very soon.

Mrs. Isida came to the hotel in the evening to ask if I would like to go to some Japanese folk dancing in the country a few miles out. I was so tired, as we had such a busy day, and I had made an appointment for the following morning to visit the *jiu-jitsu* training school by 7:00 a.m., so I reluctantly declined.

On the morning of August 18, I exited the Oriental Hotel at 6:45 a.m. and found Mrs. Isida waiting for me in the hotel lobby. We took a taxi to the famous Japanese Jiu-jitsu School, which taught an entertaining and exciting form of wrestling. We also observed fencing lessons. I asked the ages of some of the little fellows and was told that they were six and a half years old. On the way back to the hotel, we stopped in at a public kindergarten and high school to see the interior and general layout.

The next evening, I invited Mr. and Mrs. Brown to have dinner with me. We motored out to Osaka, about 40 miles from Kobe, just to get a glimpse of the city. We also drove through a busy manufacturing center of three million inhabitants. On our way back to Kobe, we stopped at a well-known hotel, Koskin Inn, and ate a very delicious dinner.

Early in the afternoon on August 18, I packed my bag and carried my carnations from the beautiful Japanese gardens so tastefully arranged with greens, and waited for my taxi. I had quite a send-off from Mrs. Isida and Mrs. Brown. Her two-year-old charge and amah, a sweet lady by the name of Madeline, came down to see me off. Even Mr. Brown dashed out of a taxi and ran aboard just a few minutes before the siren blew for visitors to go ashore to say goodbye.

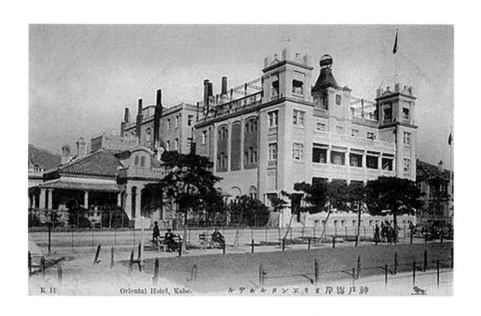

Oriental Hotel, Kobe Japan (above) and Travel Brochure (below) 1930's

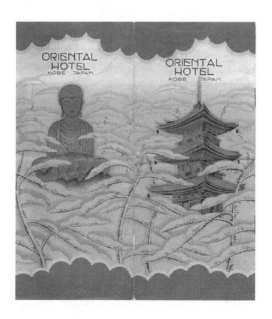

S.S. Chojo Meru: August 18, 1932

The S.S. Chojo Meru was a very nice ship and most comfortable. They had superb food with not much variety, but nothing to complain of. In fact, I was glad to get such a simple and adequate menu after the Oriental Hotel and Empress of Japan's complicated bills affair; the menu suited me much better. There were twenty people who boarded when I did and quite a few English. I sat next to the Japanese purser and an Englishman opposite end next to my right. The purser—a nice, extremely pleasant, little man—spoke a little English and felt badly when he could not answer all of the questions that were fired at him in English. He seemed very much pleased that I liked Japan and beamed and bowed every time I entered or left the dining room salon.

I met two Englishman from the British Army of Tientsin. I like done well; he said that he would come to see me in Peiping. His stepfather, Mr. Douglas decided to sail with him to China. There seemed to be a functional relationship between stepfather and son, which was rather unusual from my experience.

We enjoyed sailing through the inland sea and we spent a few hours on shore at Mojo. I was escorted by three strapping Englishman, all in tropical white attire, two of them wearing a light white helmet. The ship's captain, another pleasant Japanese man, took me into the chart room in the morning and pointed out our course to me. He said we had just escaped a typhoon. We felt just a little swell, what he called the tall end, so I think we were most fortunate. We sailed past the coast of Korea and entered the Yellow Sea.

It was hard for me to believe it would be just four weeks and three days from port to port. I had left Boston on Friday, July 22, and expected to reach Peiping on August 22. I had hoped that I could get a connection for Tientsin and Peiping. Tangku was further from paying by twenty miles, but we reached it first, and the water was too shallow to go by steamer to Tientsin.

My four-day trip from Kobe to Tientsin along the Korean coast was interesting. I saw beautiful small and large islands that were captivating.

161

I'm surprised that I heard so little of the beauty of this stretch of the voyage beforehand. The sights were filled with the simplicity of living and brought a sense of restfulness to my soul. The ships did not go up as far as Tientsin, so we first landed in China in a dirty and interesting spot called the Tangku.

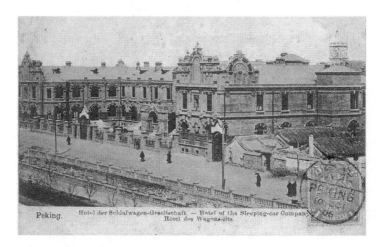

Grand Hotel des Wagons Lits (Peiping, China)

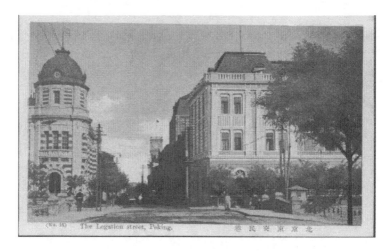

Yokohama Specie Bank on the left and the Grand Hotel des Wagons-Lits on the right

The usual thought and consideration of the Peiping University Medical College directors forestalled any inconvenience that might come from arriving in a foreign country from encountering customs by sending someone to meet me at the steamer. They handed me a little note at breakfast stating that Mr. Wang, one of the college staff from the office of the treasurer, would be awaiting me.

In consequence, I had no trouble with the customs, with not even care with my handbag.

The hospital took care of all of the tasks regarding my arrival until I carried on the final lap of destination. Mr. Wayne, my escort from the college, even brought sandwiches that we lunched upon with a warm beer.

At about 2:30 p.m. on August 22, the ship landed in Peiping. There was quite a delegation that came down to meet me at the station. Mr. Greene; Dr. Meug; Mrs. Walker, the superintendent secretary; and Miss Loh, my predecessor in the physical therapy department, all welcomed me with open arms.

I was anxious to see the hospital, but I first stopped to check into my room at the Grand Hotel des Wagons Lits in the Legation Quarter, located in the Dongcheng District directly to the east of Tiananmen Square. It was a grand hotel designed in the Flemish Gothic style. They told me several diplomats worked in the Legations area and the soldiers guarded them, so I felt very safe. I later found a sizable number of scholars, artists, and athletes lived there and were attracted by the ancient Chinese culture preserved in the city and were able to be there leisurely for very little money. Mr. Greene sent his car back for me an hour later and for the first time I drove up to the main entrance of Peiping University Medical College. It looked like the group of massive Chinese temples I had seen in photographs that were originally built as a pricey private mansion.

The college cuts quite a figure in the heart of the busy shopping section of the city. The main building was a very beautiful one built of white stone with pretty grass and a green tile roof. It was an enchanted campus of imposing buildings. Its walls were built of stone and the architecture and general style were Chinese. It also had green tiled roofs with little Chinese porcelain figures at the top of each curbing corner. There were from five to seven of the little, green porcelain figures at each corner; the figure nearest that outer side of the building was a cock, upon which was seated a little image, supposedly of an evil spirit.

Next to the building there was a green porcelain dragon. Between the mountain cock and the dragon were several little mounted figures. The Chinese people have many superstitions and stories that the evil spirit at the outside edge of the roof cannot fall off the sacred cock; the animals in between keep it from dismounting, therefore, the evil spirit cannot get past the dragon so it cannot enter the building and all is well inside.

The college buildings were arranged in a quadrangular form and architecturally pleasing to the eye. At the center of the campus stood the main building, gate, and dormitory, which was the former Manchu residence. The pathology, chemistry, and anatomy buildings—which shared a connecting corridor with BNC house— were surrounded by its administrative, registers, and treasurer's offices. The medical school was in Building D. There was also the beautiful, decorated Laura Spelman wing that was used as the nurses' lounge, duly named after John D. Rockefeller's wife.

The approach to these buildings began with a white marble stairway composed of two short flights of steps, one on either side of the marble slabs upon which were groups of handsomely carved dragons. The carved slabs were known as the "spirit stairway." The buildings were surrounded by gardens and tennis courts, which took away the institutional atmosphere.

164

The hospital's different wards were connected with the medical school by means of long runways of artistic, white stone mosaic and green tile. There were about twelve or fourteen wards; these outside mosaic tile passages joined together. The Chinese people have an innate abhorrence of hospitals, therefore, these atheistic arrangements were sound psychology decorations to help them seek care. There was a fine selection of medical books in the library, too, and a varied assortment of other literature.

Primarily, the medical school and hospital functioned for research purposes. There were approximately 200 doctors on the staff, many of who were young Chinese who had their medical training in the college, others from different schools of medicine in China; 360 beds filled the hospital and were often full.

A group of missionary people with the Qing government founded the school in 1906. They fashioned it after Johns Hopkins and in 1917, the Rockefeller Foundation assumed financial responsibility for its operations. It became the leading hospital and training center in China.

The physical department was a large and well-equipped department but I could see right away I had a lot of challenges ahead. After my visit, I found it a tremendous handicap to not be able to speak a word of Chinese. I decided at that moment I should start on a speaking lesson every day right away.

Everybody was so kind to me my first evening. They invited me to dinner at the home of the registrar, Mrs. Ferguson. We ate outdoors in a truly typical Chinese garden under the spreading willow tree. Everything was so quiet and peaceful; the gardens were all walled off in a way that there was nothing else in the world. I got to know a few of the staff and was given an overview of the how the hospital was run and left with great anticipation for starting my first day at work the next morning.

165

Later in the evening, I returned to my hotel room and slept well in my firm bed, draped with a mosquito net. The room was lovely and cozy. The furniture was made of pear rose, set against a background of Chinese calligraphy and paintings that hung on the wall.

The first few days at the hospital were like finding my way through a haze of fog. I spent as much as time as possible with Miss Loh, as she would leave the following week. She walked me through all the operations with a group of five women and three men, one whom had limited knowledge of English. Mr. Change was an earnest and conscientious lad with nurse's training and I knew he would be a godsend to me.

One week later, my predecessor, Miss Loh, left for a year special study in physical therapy at Northwestern University, Chicago. Dr. Wang, the superintendent, and Mrs. Walker kindly invited me to drive down to the station with them to see her off. I was glad to go and pleased to have had an opportunity of getting acquainted, even for a few days, with her. I liked her and felt that her attitude regarding my coming into the department had been all and more that might have been expected because of her.

Now that she had left, I was quite independent and on my own except for the interpretation of the senior male nurse, Mr. Change, a nurse in the physical therapy department. He was just as nice as could be, most helpful and so respectful. I was most fortunate.

My department assistants invited me to attend a real Chinese dinner at a local restaurant and what a welcome feast it was. I was careful as to what I ate as the food was very new to me. There was a lot of attention paid to a bowl of boiling broth in the table's center. They used another boiling kettle of water to sterilize every dish, plate, glass, and utensils.

The only eating utensils were two pairs of chopsticks, one China spoon, and one silver-plated spoon. I think the spoons must have been in my honor, but I did myself proud by only using the chopsticks. Dish after dish was brought out, each one representing another course of Chinese fare, and each tasting quite different and good to me. We must have had at least twelve or fourteen courses. I was offered beer and wine, but chose the former. The Chinese, as a people, I understand, were quite abstemious regarding alcohol beverages.

During the first month at PUMC, I reorganized the physical therapy department and treatment rooms. They had a lot of out-datedå equipment and I had to convince the board to get rid of it and buy new ones. Sadly, I had to let go of some of the personnel because they were not able to reach the level of expectation I needed them to.

I was excited at times, frustrated at other times, but motivated to do the best job I could do and make my family and comrades proud. I had to study the language every day and learned quickly that, "To get adjusted to the world, after all, the better plan—it won't adjust itself to you, for it was here way before you came."

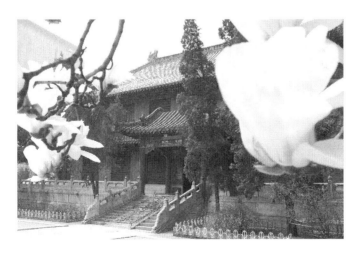

Peiping Medical University College Entrance

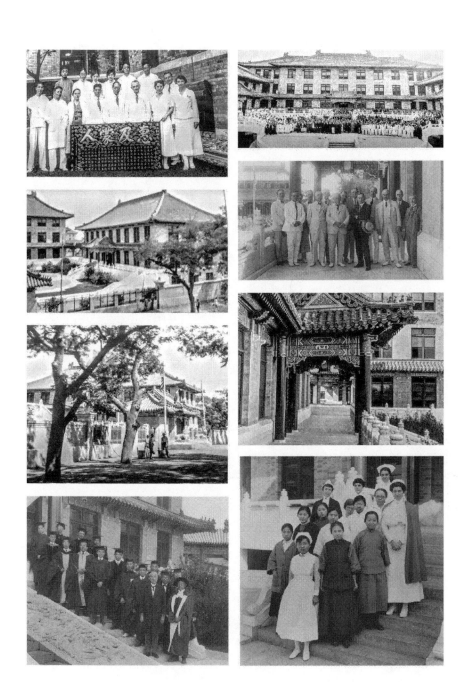

Peiping Medical College Choir, campus, doctor graduates, and nurse

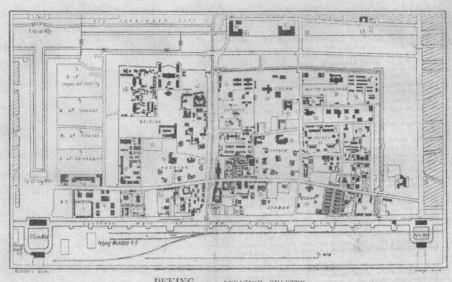

PEKING. — LEGATION QUARTER

1. Tsŏ-chin Ch'eng.
2. Tsung-jên Fu.
3. Li-pu.
4. Tu-chih-pu (formerly Hu-pu).
5. Li-pu.
6. French Hospital (St-Michel).
7. U. S. American Guard.
8. U. S. American Legation.
9. Netherlands Legation and { a, Minister,
   Guard .... { b, Guard,
10. Russian Guard.
11. Russian Legation.
12. Russo-asiatic Bank.
13. Banque de l'Indo-Chine.
14. Hôtel des Wagons-lits.
15. German Post Office.
16. Russian Post Office.
17. Hongkong and Shanghai B. C.
18. Yokohama Specie Bank.

19. Spanish Legation.
20. Japanese Guard.
21. Japanese Legation.
22. French Post Office.
23. French Legation.
24. French Guard.
25. French Catholique Church (St-Michel).
26. German Legation.
27. Belgian Legation.
28. German Guard.
29. Deutsch-Asiatische Bank.
30. Stores.
31. German Lazaret.
32. Hopkins Memorial Hospital.
33. Electric Station.
34. Imperial Maritime Customs, Residen-
    ces and Head Offices.
35. Peking Club.
36. Imperial Post of China, Secretary's
    Office.

37. Inspectorate General of Imperial Ma-
    ritime Customs.
38. Austro-Hungarian Guard.
39. Austro-Hungarian Legation.
40. Italian Legation.
41. Italian Guard.
42. British Legation { a. Minister,
                     { b. 1st Secretary,
                     { c. 2nd Secretary,
                     { d. Church.
43. British Guard.
44. Portuguese Legation.
45. Chinese Post Office.
46. Hôtel de Pekin.
47. Peking Han-k'ou R. R. Head Office.
48. International Banking Corporation.
49. Mexican Legation.
50. Telegraph Office.
51. Hôtel du Nord.

Peiping (Peking) Legation Quarters Map

11

A NEW LIFE IN CHINA

Peiping, China: December 27, 1932

Four months after I arrived in Peiping, I learned so much about the ancient northern capital. The city of Peiping was composed of three main sections: Tartar City, the Legation Quarter, and the Forbidden City. Walls surround each of the cities, with gates leading to the main thoroughfares. The walls of the Tartar City were twice as high as those of other Chinese cities. The enchanted city is located in the north, and older part, of Peiping.

The Legation Quarter occupies the southern wall of Tartar City between Chien Men and Hats Men. They set aside the area after the Boxer Uprising in 1900. Just outside the window of the hotel in which I lived was Watergate, through which the American troops entered to the relief of the beleaguered legations. The fairly broad and paved streets with several open gardens and boulevard made for pleasant daily walks.

My living quarters were charming, with a sitting room, bedroom, and bathroom. The two hotels, which catered to the Western trade, mine being the less pretentious of the two, was generally more comfortable and had the better cuisine. The manager, a Londoner, had an assistant who was Swiss, which created a good combination of hospitality. They were calm, kind, and most accommodating, and made me feel very at home at the hotel.

171

When I arrived to Peiping in August, the weather was blistering hot, along with a fair amount of rainfall in the early part of September, which I was told was rather unusual. Heavy rainfall occurred during July and the early part of August. On the whole, I considered it a remarkably beautiful autumn. The only thing I found to my distaste was the most disagreeable feature of the city—the many dust storms.

I had not experienced a bad fall season, but had walked in one or two fairly good storms. The wind blew with such velocity that the dust almost blinded you and the *hutongs* are set up haphazardly upon unpaved, dusty lanes. I will let you imagine what crazy storms do under these conditions.

The Forbidden City, or Imperial City, had been the one time residential section of the Emperor and his court. It opened to the public and some of the old beautiful buildings had been made into public museums. The Forbidden City's parks and palaces exhibited how the royal people in their heyday spent their time. The area must have been resplendent but showed its wear and tear of the years. Sadly, its remains are rather heart breaking to take in. The beautiful green tile roofs had weeds driving in between the tiles and much broken plaster on the outside of the building and courtyards.

They named the shops after the merchandise that their vendors sold, such as jade, brass, silver, or lanterns. In some of them, old treasures were stored away in dirty old rooms littered with barrels and boxes. Many of the treasures were hundreds of years old. The Chinese shops stayed open until late at night. In the Chinese section, much of the shopping was done on the pavement in front of the respective shops. Chinese policeman stood at various crossroads and carried a little black-and-white-striped stick, rather authoritatively and sometimes, with the most amusing action, they suddenly thrust their sticks out, striking rickshaw boys or chauffeurs or bicyclers.

172

They used donkeys or camels to carry their burdens, from articles of furniture to the morning vegetables and meat supplies.

I thoroughly enjoyed nightlife on the Peiping streets. It was fascinating when comfortably snuggled in the rickshaw under a robe to travel along the bustling streets at night. Each rickshaw had a little old-fashioned candle lantern on both sides, and bicycles were decorously lighted by means of parchment lanterns dangling from the handlebars. Many of the shops had similar lanterns hanging from their doorways. Each one had a jet oil burner or candle lantern not uncommonly seen.

I became interested in my work and saw quite a possibility for research in one of two branches. Between my daily works, a Chinese lesson each day, and my social life, I did not experience one dull moment. It was my privilege after a couple of months to visit Cheeloo University in Jinjin, China. The United Missionary Medical School and hospital were in the Shantung District is some 300 miles south of Peiping. I visited for a few days and enjoyed the opportunity of seeing something of the country and how another medical school hospital operated.

After a few months, PUMC was exceptionally well provided for. The physiotherapy department had good equipment and as the demand for more became necessary, I anticipated more support would be forthcoming. I trained six assistants, three male nurses, and three women—all Chinese. My first assistant, a young Chinese male nurse, was a splendid type of a young man—earnest, efficient, and spoke English well.

In the physical therapy department, we took care of the hospital patients in the morning and our visiting patients in the afternoon. I gave a course of lectures to the staff doctors, who knew little about our profession but were anxious to know more. I also had a group of postgraduate nurses who were sent by their respective hospitals from different parts of China for special instruction and observation.

173

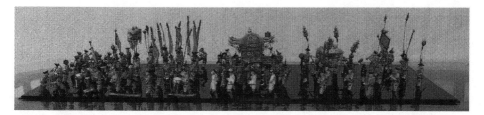

Chinese Funeral March

It is an interesting and amusing experience for a foreigner to attend a Chinese performance. One of the most fascinating sights when I walked to work at PUMC each day was observing the many funeral processions. I sometimes wondered if anyone was left in China, one sees so many funerals.

To counterbalance these funeral demonstrations, they also had many wonderful wedding processions, the latter not nearly as pretentious. The length of the funeral procession and a number of bearers for each coffin indicated the rank of the deceased. The mourners created magnificent replicas of the deceased's most treasured possessions and mementos that are constructed cleverly of bamboo and paper and carried to be burned at the grave. The higher their station in life, the more articles carried. Therefore, a person of great wealth and consequence had numerous offerings carried in the funeral procession.

All the men and small boys marched in the procession extravagantly dressed in robes of bright green and scarlet with much embroidery. Some wore a headdress that looked to the entire world like a lampshade and some carried white plumes—a heart-warming sight.

The banging of the drums and cymbals, not to mention the strange sounds that came forth from the trumpet blowers, made one realize what ceremony funeral possessions play in the hearts of Chinese people. On the top of the coffin they placed a handsomely embroidered scarlet robe. The women mourners rode in an old-fashioned-looking cab drawn by mules and wore white only.

174

The funeral processions parade route stretched a quarter to a mile. In the country, it's common sights are mounds of earth right in the center of the field adjacent to the houses. The piles of soil are the family burial grounds.

The Chinese people had a most unusual spirit of service. The rickshaw boys and amahs, especially, seemed to almost anticipate one's wishes and express the quality—the joy of service—which is so rare in the Western world. There is something delightfully natural and naïve about the average servant class, so I rather imagined it is true of the Chinese character in general. Of course, my experience had been limited more or less to the northern ones. They are often frank about perfectly natural things and childishly curious about everybody's business. They had no Western business intellect, and a sense of urgency and time never seemed to enter their way of thinking.

I had an amusing little incident happen to me one day in one of the the Chinese shops. Upon wrapping up a few small purchases, the clerk mistakenly omitted one item from the package. The next day, I sent my rickshaw boy back with a little note asking that they give him the small piece that had been forgotten by accident. My rickshaw boy returned with a card from the owner of the shop, upon which was printed his name and written beneath, your letter received. The following day, my very small purchase arrived at the college by two special messengers. The shopkeepers are such trusting souls; one could almost carry away the whole shop in exchange for signing a piece of paper even if they have never seen you before.

My life in Peiping, in many ways, was very different from the life I lived in the Western world. There were no theaters, but the social element, especially among the members of the different groups, was much busier. There was a good deal of social activity going on all the time. I also enjoyed delightful concerts at which distinguished artists appeared from time to time.

175

I had created a lovely two-bedroom home, which was beautifully decorated with the beloved Chinese furniture and ornaments I had been collecting. I took great pride in planning and nurturing my delightful garden. I grew African marigolds, large yellow daisies, and yellow and orange lilies. My outdoor courtyard took on a blaze of color when the sun shone upon it. It was glorious to look at.

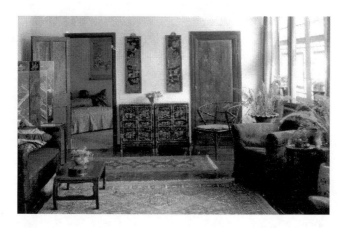

Living room of her home (above) and Christmas card photo in front of her gardens in Peiping, China (below)

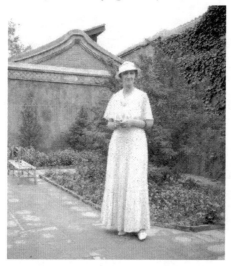

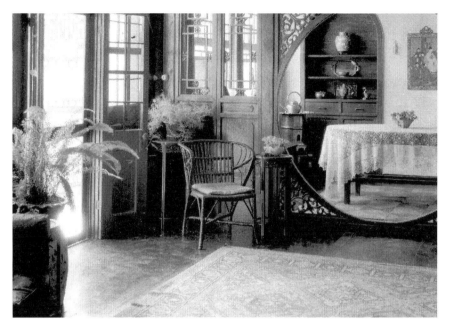

Moon shaped entry to dining room of home in Peiping, China

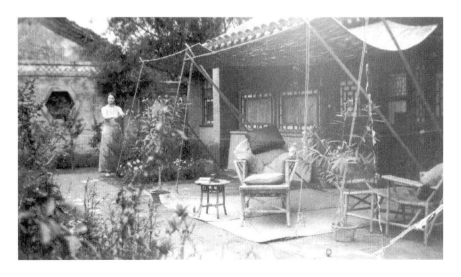

Mary in back yard and garden of her home in Peiping, China

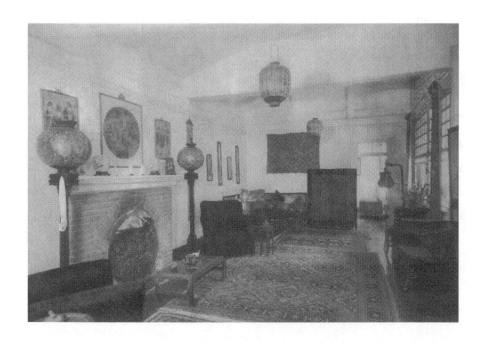

Living room of her home in Peiping, China

It had taken me two years to be able to speak the Chinese language well. I felt confident enough to take some weekend trips to see more of the country. In the fall, I spent a few interesting weekends in the country at the Summer Palace, which is within a radius of twenty miles of the city. It had been an imperial garden in the Qing dynasty and was now open to the public and surrounded by very beautiful gardens, ponds, and parks. It was very cold when I visited, no snowfall, but a sufficient frost allowed for ice-skating in January and February.

The Emperor and his court visited the palace in the summer, but the old empress dowager preferred staying there instead of the winter palace in the Forbidden City. She liked it so well that she used to go to the hills early in the spring and stay late into the autumn. There was plenty of opportunity for climbing in that section of the country and from the top of the hills one got an excellent view of the beauty of China.

One evening, one of my co-workers invited me to a dinner party in the heart of the west city where few, if any, foreigners live, in a beautiful old Chinese house. The country's houses consist of rooms built around a courtyard. This particular courtyard offered a variety of ancient trees in excellent condition. In the center of the courtyard there was a grand fountain and a vast number of flowers, that were changed accordingly to season, and quite a few flowering shrubs. Little red lanterns suspended from the shrubs were the only form of lighting.

My host, Dr. Grabean, a writer and scientist of some repute, had invited quite an unusual group of guests for the evening. There was an archaeologist, a professor of anatomy, a botanist, an astronomer, one of our PUMC professors and head of the surgical division, and the general manager of an American tobacco company, whose wife

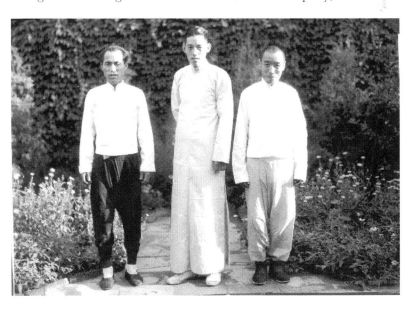

Houseboys who worked in Mary's home in Peiping, China

179

was also present. This lady was an artist; another of the ladies was a journalist. As I looked around the room, I couldn't believe each one of us was a real person at a party in China.

There were sixteen guests. We met first in the courtyard, later going under the outdoor cover with windows and door open, basking in the beauty of the evening with all its quiet restful sounds. Then the party moved inside. They served our delightful meal under candlelight; two handsome silver candelabra having very tall Chinese red candles in each. Table effects were in the same silver and lacquer red. On a long, black table, colorful Chinese-designed dishes looked particularly elegant.

We exchanged fascinating stories, which I found intensely interesting. I discovered several of the group had taken trips together in different parts of the world. The conversation at no time was trivial; sometimes it was scintillating, added with a galaxy of intellect and humor.

We rose from the table at 10:20 p.m. and left immediately as martial law was in effect. There had been a long, simmering conflict with Japan, and China would rear its ugly head once again, which meant we were about to see it explode again. We needed to leave because Dr. Louck's chauffeur stood-in with the Chinese police, where we could go to the city gates even at that hour. I wish I could express more adequately the many priceless experiences I had in China. So many of these accounts! I shall never forget the rare, rich, and treasured memories.

One such trip I took was to the sacred mountain, Mount Taishan and Chu Fou. The quaint little village in which Confucius lived and where he is buried, 5,300 feet above sea level. There were 6,300 stone steps that visitors must climb before they reach the summit, making it quite an adventure. Every spring there were many pilgrims who made the trip; some climbed many of the stone stairs on hands and knees. When they reached the temple at the summit and made their monastery contributions, they were considered to have an absolution of past sins and were ensured future protection for the next reincarnation. Every devout Taoist takes this astounding journey at least once in their lifetime.

We saw old men and women, the latter with bound feet, making the trip. In every party, each hired a sedan chair and three coolie carriers to make the journey. We started on the journey at one o'clock midday having traveled overnight by train from Peiping to Tian Tou. We reached the summit by 7:00 p.m., just in time to see the sunset over the tops of the surrounding mountains.

We slept on hard boards in a temple at the feet of the Buddha and were up before 5:00 a.m. to see the sunrise. On the return trip the views were magnificent with the gorges covered with hanging fresh and green foliage. We passed many smaller temples and saw the native men, women, and children in their crude, primitive mud huts with strong roofs. I assumed, by the way they were dressed, they were all Taoist. The men had part of their heads shorn with peculiar-looking tufts of hair; some also had a long plait.

We had breakfast at 6:00 a.m. and started down the mountain soon after. We reached the foot around noontime. I looked forward to a long bath, which would now seem like a luxury, and a much needed simple, wholesome meal I am sure would have seemed better than any served at the Ritz-Carlton we had eaten.

The train trip to Chu Fou, the home of Confucius, takes about two or three hours to the station. The interesting part is when the station is left behind, you still have to travel on a quaint covered donkey cart, known as a "Peiping cart," across fields and along a sandy stretch that leads to the village itself, which was six miles away. We slept that night in a bare room in the courtyard of the Mission Station, arose early and breakfast was served in the courtyard before we visited the picturesque Temple of Confucius. We then saw the cemetery where we noticed they buried the son, grandson,

181

and Confucius. By 4:00 p.m. we were again on the northbound train before noonday and arrived in Peiping.

It was a rare long weekend away from Thursday to Monday, with Friday being a Chinese holiday. We saw some never-to-be-forgotten sites, had congenial companionship, and decided that a real good night's sleep was what we needed most of all. That trip was exactly two weeks away from the real tension of the Sino-Japanese trouble and was keenly felt in Peiping. When we returned, we were told 500 first class tickets for passage on a ship out of Peiping had been sold in one week and I couldn't quite believe it.

PART FOUR
1933-1943

12

AN AMERICAN APPRECIATES THE CHINESE WAY OF LIFE

Peiping Union Medical College, China: May 12, 1933

O ne morning in the middle of May 1933, I awakened from a deep sleep by a whizzing sound above the house, immediately followed by what I thought was a knock on my bedroom door. I mumbled something rather sleepily, and again there was a knock at my door. This time I distinctly called out, "Come in," thinking it was the houseboy bringing the early morning water to drink, but I received no reply.

I looked at my watch and found it to be six o'clock in the morning, just an hour earlier than the usual time I woke up. There was little time to speculate the where and wherefores because one knock followed another so fast and left no doubt that the Japanese were flying above our city and sending skyrockets into the heavens. I opened the door and found that the only people in the house were two ladies in the hallway and the servants outside. We looked at one another and said, "Well, they have come." One of our houseboys ran up to us with the paper in his hand that had been dropped from one of the Japanese airplanes a few minutes before. The enemy printed the following note in Chinese script: *Why follow Chiang Kai-shek, he has nothing to give you. He has no guns, we have big guns. We were on our way.*

I thought to myself, *how polite our Japanese neighbors are distributing calling cards today, early in the morning*. I packed up my small valuables into my pillbox thinking, *blessed be nothing*, and scurried my way to the college. Everybody was aware and surprisingly no one felt a great, apparent alarm and our patients came and went as usual.

It is important to keep a good attitude, as the fear of the unknown would become unbearable. I knew for years that the Japanese had an imperialist policy to expand its political influence and military presence in China, and to secure access to raw materials, food, and labor. The Manchurian Incident, commonly known as the Mukden Incident, in 1931 reignited the beginning of the turmoil between China and Japan. The Mukden Incident was an explosion staged by rogue military officials in an attempt to justify the Japanese invasion of North-eastern China, known as Manchuria. They had continued small engagements and incidents since that time.

Seven days had passed since the Japanese airplanes flew above the city. Ever since that time, every sound we heard was interpreted as the possible invasion of the Japanese into the city of Peiping. It became clear the Japanese wanted to take over the city. The poor Chinese from the surrounding small towns and villages arrived into the city in droves. For several missions' stations in Honon nearby had consignments of refugees. The first group who arrived were around 200 men, women, and children. Their worldly effects stacked on the backs of mules and oxen—carrying crude pieces of furniture, bedding, and sacks of wheat.

The area in which I lived was exquisite, with its well-kept lawns and old trees, but at this time they blocked the entrance in order to provide stables for the refugees, mules, and their oxen. They housed the people en masse in the neighbourhood church. All the food vendors were doing a lively trade because all the Chinese dishes sold out at almost all the street corners.

188

The Salvation Army worked hard helping to feed many of the refugees. It was not the Japanese we were really afraid of, but rather the large groups of Chinese soldiers who were escaping Jehol and the northern provinces and then retreating into Peiping. That was when the people became afraid. Looting seemed to be a legitimate part of Chinese warfare. The soldiers, or many of them, had been poorly paid and badly fed for months. Therefore, they thought nothing of helping themselves to anything they needed en route to their destination.

Many of our coolies at the college had to leave their homes so that the soldiers had a place to live. There was no such thing in Chinese warfare as billeting team in family homes, like with the families in France and England during the Great War. Here, the soldiers occupied any house they decided they wanted and as many of them as they decided they needed, and the Chinese have to get out.

We had thousands of Chinese soldiers in the city because we suspected there would be a considerable resistance offered when the Japanese entered the city. We never knew the day nor the hour they would come. Each day we heard Japanese planes overhead and the unknowing of what was going to happen seemed insufferable at times.

One day, the Chinese soldiers who were guarding the wall, just a stone's throw from where I lived, fired into the air, foolishly thinking they could hit a Japanese plane. Instead, the shot broke not far in the air, but onto the ground, badly wounding two innocent laborers who were immediately brought into the college hospital.

There was surely no doubt now about the Japanese invading Peiping. Part of me wished they would come and get it over with so that the suspense and irresolute feelings would be over.

189

We lived at the time in fear. Not knowing was much more heart wrenching than what we thought when the Japanese finally came. At that time, most of the Chinese had given up hope, and more or less resigned that Japanese would takeover and felt helpless under the circumstances.

Tanggu Truce: May 22, 1933

The fear and uncertainty had been building tension in everyone's psyche day by day. Each day we awoke with Japanese airplanes flying overhead. In preparation of a possible attack on our city, people filled thousands of sacks with sand and dirt; the latter was the easiest thing to find in Peiping. They placed the weighted sandbags at the important junctions of all the big streets and the larger and more important hutongs.

At the time I did not understand the principle of the scheme, but now know the Chinese used these anchors piled high to create a kind of barrage, in an attempt to save a big thoroughfare. It seemed rather futile to me at the time because I imagined that the Japanese would use an entirely different method of attack. They knew the city well and had no sympathy for the Chinese people.

While we paced the halls anxiously, still expecting something bad to happen at any minute, I understood from the reports that the Japanese troops were located only a few miles outside the city. In anticipation of the siege, the housekeepers only bought staples and necessities as prices were soaring.

Each day, refugees flocked from neighbouring places into the city, along with the 30,000 troops already crowded in the city. They told me several hundred of our wounded soldiers had been taken further south in trucks; many of the patients having physiotherapy treatments and I was sorry to have them leave.

A most tragic part was the quantity of youngsters that had lost their parents from Japanese attacks, and their homes and personal effects being shattered and destroyed. We had several youngsters who

190

came to us for treatment. One dear little fellow, only eight years old, shared his sad story with us. He was playing in his own courtyard inside the Great Wall south of Kupaiku, about 90 miles from Peiping. The local policeman told him he had better go indoors because Japanese planes were flying overhead. He had just gotten inside the house when a bomb dropped onto his home. His father and mother died right before his eyes. His right hand had been badly mutilated; one of his eyes and cheeks gashed open. It is by sheer fate he survived.

The soldiers carried the boy all the way south to Peiping in their arms, wounded though they were. At times, they rode in old broken-down carts, and they finished the journey of 90 miles by rickshaw. The little fellow was first taken to the base hospital and then transferred to us.

When I visited him for the last time he had been making an excellent recovery. His cheek had healed and the operation on his hand had worked wonders. One was able to keep up their faith when visiting him because he was such a happy and approachable youngster, despite his pain and loss. Whenever he saw me coming into the ward, he would reach his little hand out to mine in gratitude.

It just wrung people's hearts to see such tragic sites, and while many of them were similar, many, it's sad to say, were much worse. One little girl lost both her hands completely. It's hard to share the details, but I feel I must tell her story. Do you know what that no-handed, eight-year-old girl answered when one of our staff asked her the following question: "What will you do when you leave here?" The girl replied, "Go back to where I came." Another nurse asked, "Well, what will you do if the Japanese bomb your home again?" To which she answered, "I suppose I should follow my mother." Both her mother and father had been killed. *Don't you call that a neighbourhood philosophy at only eight years of age?* I do. She made that reply without a qualm, in fact, with a peaceful smile on her face—certainly without the slightest sign of fear.

191

Mass groups of Chinese soldiers, without restraint, hoarded and looted the city. I was surprised at this because the Chinese people are most dear and generous in spirit. It may be the soldiers' last hope after hearing about the Chinese and Japanese representatives meeting in Tanggu, Tianjin to negotiate an end of the conflict, by creating a demilitarized zone extending 100 kilometers south of the Great Wall, which up until that time, the Japanese had been prohibited from entering.

On June 1, we were all happy and relieved to hear the latest war news. Whatever the military armistice may have meant, the government was supposedly going through the process of establishing one with the Japanese, which we learned from the Peiping Chronicle.

In any case, the crippling atmosphere of fear had been cleared for the present. For how long a time it would last, we did not know, nor did anyone else. Everyone at the college continued to move forward, day by day, with our mission to assist and help as many people as we could. We kept a sense of hope, due in part to experiencing an usually early summer that year. The daily rainfall helped the green grass and flowers spring into brilliant freshness. Even in the tragedy and darkness of war, there was a glorious glow— showing of pink, red, and white peonies—as I walked home each day from the college.

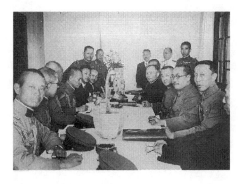

The Tanggu Truce negotiations to end conflict

192

A Chinese Wedding:
January 14, 1934

On a chilly winter Sunday in January 1934, a special wedding took place in Peiping. These happy events were common enough during the weekends, but this wedding was unique because the bride was a nurse who worked in my department and she asked me to be a special guest at the wedding. I had never been to a Chinese wedding and was so taken aback by it beauty and neighbour. The bride was a young and beautiful pure Chinese type, who was quiet and reserved with a responsive nature reflected in her expression.

A week or two before the event, I received an invitation to the wedding. The Chinese wedding color is most often red and they had printed the invitation on bright red, heavy paper. The size, four inches wide by six inches long, was pressed into a double sheet. Upon opening the envelope, on the right-hand side of the right-hand sheet in gold letters were the bride and bridegroom's names printed in Chinese characters.

Chinese books are printed from the back to the front, so the name to whom the invitation was for was on the backside, just the reverse way from the Western style. The text was inscribed in Chinese characters, but the black ink on the outer side was printed in gold and told the address of the bride's home, or the hotel at which her friends would receive her the morning of the wedding. On the left side of the sheet listed the meeting at the groom's house in gold characters. Facing on the left-hand sheet were two very large gold characters that signified long life and happiness.

The groom, also young and well educated, belonged to an old and much respected Chinese family. Both the parents of the bride and bridegroom had come under little influence of the Western world. In each case, the mothers had Chinese bound feet from the old school customs.

193

The bride requested that I be ready to start at eleven o'clock in the morning and she would have someone drive me to her home. Shortly after eleven, the bridesmaid stood at my front door in a pretty blue silk *ishang* with peach-colored flowers in her hair. The charming little lady stood before me and, although she could not speak English, her gracious manner intimated even more genial than words of cordial welcome to a foreign guest.

We drove along the narrow hutung streets resembling lanes and into one of the main shopping streets. Chinese shops were open every day of the week, in fact Sundays were their most crowded shopping days. We passed the big covered market, known as the "East Market," and saw a morning crowd of shoppers, where everything could be purchased from hats to shoes. The more delightful edibles could also be obtained in this market, such as delectable tidbits like glazed nuts, candies, and fruits—the latter being piled high on open stores outside the shops. Fear of exposing either food or individuals to germs in the middle of the war were the least of the worries in China.

At the entrance to the market, there were rickshaws with their indispensable appendices, "*la-chush-ti*" the rickshaw boy, bound into the crowds the size of a football game. A sea of honeybees all eager to earn a copper or two, a small income may have been the only thing between them and starvation. No wonder there was insistent cries of "*yao pu yao*" or "want or not want a rickshaw."

We reached our destination, a smaller Chinese hotel of which Peiping acknowledges some 6,000 people or more. Weddings in Peiping are celebrated in hotels rather than at the homes of the participants. The bride's mother, in this case, hired a small hotel so that only the bride's parents, family members, and friends gathered before the ceremony.

194

We entered from the main thoroughfare, which happened to be one on the wide city streets, through an old but latticed gate, onto the first courtyard, passing by a "demon screen" made of wood or plaster. Chinese characters are painted over carvings on decorative screens, denoting that the good spirits are welcome. Screens are placed at the entrances to keep out the evil spirits. Demon screens may be seen outside almost all the large or public buildings, temples, hotels, or private residences.

Next, we went into the second courtyard where the little brid cordially greeted each guest. Having a father, brother, and an aged mother made it necessary for the bride to spend most of her time looking out for her guests. The male guests were naturally separated from the women. The bride's mother offered many bows and Chinese words of greeting as she welcomed the guests. She wore a dark green silk ishang—a dress that is a long, plain, padded coat with a high collar with long sleeves, worn alike by Chinese men and women. The bride looked beautiful in a light, pale green silk ishang with slippers to match. I could see under the long high slit at the side of the dress a pair of lovely green silk trousers to match.

Upon entering the house, each guest was given a large red paper chrysanthemum to pin onto their dresses to signify that we were guests at the wedding. Several dozen women and many children gathered in the large room, all wearing their best ishang with the red paper flowers. The medley of color looked as artistic and colourful.

It was a clear, cold, crisp day and fortunately with little wind, but the temperature registered between freezing point and zero. Two large Chinese stoves inside the room on both sides of the door were the only means of heating the large room. The sun streaming into the courtyard area helped to make the room more cozy and comfortable.

195

I found it interesting to see all the happy faces and hear the greetings exchanged from friend to friend. Five tables were set up in the middle of the room and covered with red tablecloths. The table to which I was invited to sit had the brides more intimate school friends only, a nice interesting group of young people. I was the only Westerner present and seemed to be treated as a guest of honor. They invited me to sit at the center table and with great error; I immediately took the place of privilege, and then I noticed that they asked the next guest to be seated at my right and she voraciously declined for at least four or five minutes. Only then did I realize what a faux pas I had made.

Ten guests sat around each table while the bride and her mother passed among their guests encouraging them to eat and drink, but neither ate nor drank themselves. They served a grand Chinese feast in large bowls set in the middle of each table. They gave a small individual plate to each guest to share a numerous variety of Chinese food to be eaten. Besides the tiny plate, each guest was provided with a porcelain spoon, a pair of ivory chopsticks, and a tiny wine cup.

A Chinese teapot with hot Chinese rice wine was poured into each of the little teacups, and there was a vigilant watch to see when the wine in the cup was emptied, at which time it was replenished. Each person stretched forth with their own chopsticks to help themselves from the center bowl.

When we first sat down, there were trays of sugar nuts, candied fruit, cold chicken, cold ham, and a unique thousand-year-old dish. The dish consisted of eggs preserved in salt and spices, and then covered with a mixture of mud and straw for 40 days. They brought it forth and sliced it to look like a strong coffee jelly. In color, it was dark greenish-brown. Next was steaming hot food, like small pieces of meat cooked with bamboo sprouts, hot mushrooms and diced pork in bean sauce, then a freshly baked dish in sour, sweet sauce. Next, chicken velvet was offered, which is a delicious way of cooking only the white chicken breasts in addition to Peiping duck in a flat Wheaton pancake.

In addition, they served hot, Chinese-steamed, white wheat bread with the soup and rice. A large bowl of soup made of shark fins, which are a rare delicacy, followed by cabbage soup, and lastly a sweet concoction known as orange and walnut soup.

The actual feast probably lasted an hour after which only the more intimate friends of the bride followed her into the bridal chamber, which she would later emerge from as a resplendent bride, ready to enter the gorgeously-decked bridal sedan chair that every Chinese bride carried to the home of her future husband.

I found it amusing to see the interest that the young girls displayed in the different things of the bridal trousseau: the veil, the embroidery of the dress, and the shoes. I could see a good deal of them poked fun at the little bride, for her blushes were not spared in the least. After a half an hour or so, the girls ended their intimacies and fun, and the friends retired in order that the bride might adorn herself in all her finery that had been so meticulously planned for this occasion. Naturally, I also expected to leave at the time and made my ado when the bride unexpectedly asked me to stay while she dressed.

Imagine my delight at such an opportunity. No other person was present in the room but the bride, her dresser, and the bridesmaids. They lathered the bride's face with lotions, creams, rouge, and powder as if in an American beauty parlor. I had a very liberal education of beauty culture but I must admit that it was a revelation to me to see what they could accomplish, as she looked ravishingly beautiful.

Next, they put the exquisite handmade undergarments and wedding dress on her. The long trousers made of soft pale green satin were handsomely embroidered in pink. The wedding garment was fashioned in the same soft pink color with similar embroidery.

197

The dress cut as a typical Chinese ishang with a high collar and long sleeves and a sled at each of the sides of the shirt, almost   up to the knees. This made it impossible to see the handsomely embroidered trousers. The slippers were also embroidered to match, and Cinderella herself could have not shown a prettier little foot than my little Chinese bride.

A long lace net wedding veil draped most gracefully around her head. It took over an hour to dress the bride, and was one of the most interesting and illuminating hours of my life. They added a wreath of orange blossoms to hold the veil, and long dripping crystal earrings were the last touch. The bride carried a beautiful bouquet of tiny pink roses from which long ribbon streamers draped and trailed behind her. The bridesmaids also looked lovely in their satin peach-colored ishangs, similar in style to that of the bride.

While the bride was getting dressed, the groom came to pay his respects to her mother. This consists of many *kowtows*. The *kowtowing* is quite a ceremony and a very important part of a Chinese wedding. Shortly thereafter, he left to return to his family's home. The boom, boom of the drums and the bleeding of the trumpets made us aware that the band had arrived to escort the bride and her friends to the groom's house. We stepped into the large room where they asked their guests to assemble. Four of the dearest little Chinese youngsters of about four years old dressed in bright red ishangs waited to proceed the bride carrying flower baskets and the long trail in a veil.

The band's thunderous music played. There were probably 25 musicians with trumpets and drums lined up in a formation playing Chinese wedding music for such an occasion. Never shall I forget watching the bride in all of her neighbour enter the sedan chair waiting for her outside the outer gate, drawn by two large, yellow horses bedecked with flowers.

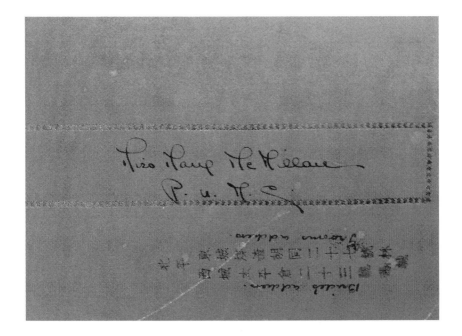

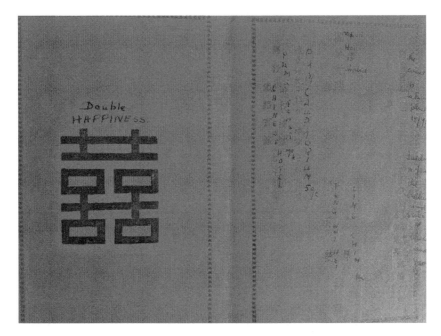

Double
HAPPINESS

Mary McMillan's Chinese wedding invitation

There was a rather touching little scene when the bride said farewell to her mother and childhood home, both women crying tears of sadness and joy. There is much more pathos when a daughter is leaving her mother in China than there is with the parting of the Western mother and daughter at such a time because the daughter from the time of her marriage now belongs to her husband and her husband's family. She will now be much more the daughter of her mother-in-law after her marriage than she will be the daughter of her own mother.

Immediately followed by the bride's chair in a Chinese carriage, I was invited to ride along with the bridesmaid in the first carriage. The whole experience was fascinating to me and I was touched at being so much a part of this oriental wedding. The precession began, the band in front all finely red coated with gold braided bands. The men immediately followed the bride's chair and other carriages. For the first time in my life I was seated in one of the queen's Chinese carriages. Inside the top of the side of the carriage, a white drapery and quaint little curtains hung in the windows. The coachman was a funny little Chinese man dressed in a uniform and seated on the top. Another man stood away, up at the back, and helped the guests into the carriage. The poor old bedecked horses looked as if they might have seen better days for all their finery.

The groom's parents had engaged a much larger hotel than the bride's mother. Hundreds of people, friends of the groom and his parents, gathered in the main banquet room. The father and mother of the groom, and even the groom himself, greeted me cordially. He was a nice-looking young man, probably around 25, the groom younger than the bride, which is often the case in Chinese marriages. He was fairly tall and wore an embossed long blue silk ishang with a separate little black corded silk jacket bound around a black silk braid. He had a flat red flower pinned to his jacket, which all the immediate family of both bride and bridegroom were wearing.

I didn't know when I'd seen such a large group of people assembled at a private ceremony; between the bride and the groom's friends there were no less than 400 or 500 people. They asked each guest to write their names in the wedding book when they arrived.

The bride and bridesmaids had quite a flourished entrance. The bride would have been crushed except for some ushers who protected her. In order to save her from the crowd's poking and the volley of confetti flying through the air, a large black sheet was held over the bride and bridesmaids soon after they entered the first courtyard. The groom himself preceded the shrouded procession. The room in which the marriage ceremony took place had a long table, upon which yellow parchment sheets were placed side- by-side. Setting on the table were the marriage rites of both bride and bridegroom written on yellow parchment paper. The vows were very elaborately displayed on a satin background and canopy up overhead upon which the Chinese characters stitched in gold thread signifying long life and happiness.

A small chamber with the Chinese *chuong*, a bed with a red canopy and a red cover awaited the bride and groom before the ceremony. The young people were very noisy, calling and singing, in fact, making it impossible for the marriage rites to take place.

The two Chinese marriage officials sat on each other's chair beneath the canopy waiting for the bride and groom. The chief usher, several times, stood at the top of a flight of stairs and entreated the young people to be quiet. The ceremony began and an old man read certain portions from a Chinese book before another official took over part two of the procedure. After they finished, they asked the young couple to place their signatures on a scroll and a seal was attached. The first bridesmaid also attached her signature, as did the matchmaker.

201

After this, the mother of the bride kowtowed, the married couple made their first kowtow to his parents, then to her parents, and the ceremony ended.

The guests were seated in an enormous courtyard around tables spread for the marriage feast. My stomach was still full after the morning bridal meal; I doubted I could eat another bite, so I made my way through the crowd and thanked my host and hostess. I had hoped I could leave but could not escape the bridegroom's eagle eye, for he came forward and tried to persuade me to remain for the second feast. I shook hands with him and told him that I must respectfully take my departure as I had another engagement. He very kindly escorted me to one of the Chinese carriages waiting outside and made sure that I was comfortably seated. The directions were given to the driver to take me back to my home. I left at five o'clock, but the festivities went on for another five to six hours because a Chinese wedding is one of the biggest events of one's lifetime.

Life in the Orient took on a variety of hues for me. For a majority of Westerners, it was never humdrum. My thoughts often strayed from China and spanned the gulf that divides to my family in America. Yet, I pulled more friends into my life, day by day, by the interesting, old, and ever-changing world. I now felt I somehow belonged to in China.

After all, we humans are merely moving electrons and are now considered almost a market commodity to the whole world. Why can't our thoughts also be transmitted on those same waves? I like to think that after all, there are no barriers, but rather that our thoughts are things with airy wings swifter than carrier doves, and perchance, before many moons have waned, we will be able to see and do here where those whom we care about and who care about us, even though both land and sea separate our physical bodies, we will find a way to connect.

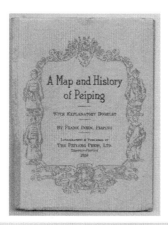

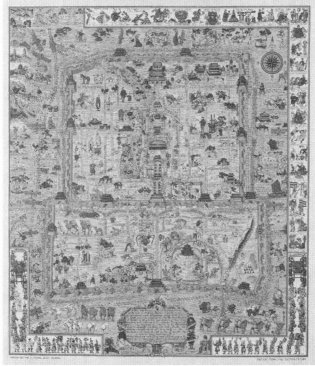

A Map and History of Peiping 1936

Peiping Union Medical College Break

September 25, 1934

In the fall of 1934, I took time off to travel and see a glimpse of the interior parts of China. My traveling companion would be my neighbour at PUMC, the nurse in charge of occupational therapy. Miss Tirzah Bullington—a native of the state of Texas— had lived, for the past two years, in more countries on the continent of Europe than one can count on one hand, as well as in Honolulu. She was a regular nomad and made an excellent traveling companion. We left Peiping on a midnight train and spent the first night lying on a thin mattress bound around a wooden slate. It was a terrifically hot night, but we were fortunate to have the small compartment to ourselves. One must not only be supplied with food and drink when traveling into the interior of the country, but also have bedding, towels, a few eating utensils, cutlery, and other incidentals.

Each of us were provided with the bare necessities when we reached the junction on the border of Shanxi province around eight o'clock the following morning and had to change trains. A narrow- gauge railway with its small engine was necessary to make the ascent of several thousand feet into the mountains of Sansai.

We gazed out upon the glorious scenery and were in awe of its stunning fertile valleys and terraced mountainsides. The houses fashioned by cutting caves out from the side of the mountains. The dwellings made entirely of terracotta mud. The cave dwellers cultivated the good earth and seemed to have plenty of progress in return. We passed many such villages. The houses resembled the adobe cave dwellings in New Mexico.

The mountains, streams of running water, and rich agriculture grounds were different from the flat drab country in the Hopsi province, along the northern coast where the crops grew rather poorly and none too plentiful. Although there were acres of irrigated rice paddies from which the natives produced a bare living existence, the rest of the country consisted of flat, barren planes.

In Shanxi province we saw a variety of crops such as millet, wheat, corn, and kaoliang. The four principal crops that feed China's 400 million people. I found it interesting to see the pomegranate trees, grapevines, and groves of walnut and date trees, in addition to many other fruit trees in great perfusion.

We reached Taiyuanfu, the capital of Shanxi, at about 7:00 p.m. The beautiful country through which we passed offered many new curiosities. Our Chinese traveling companion spoke not a word of English, but seemed amused by his Western traveling companions. We sipped tea together and exchanged courtesies. By the time we had reached our destination, he befriended us to the extent of tending to the unloading of our trappings and suggested that he hire rickshaws for us.

Just as we had expected, we found Mr. Yen waiting at the station for us. He was the nephew of Marshal Yen Han Hun, the governor of Shanxi province. The governor had no son, therefore his nephew was considered like a son and a very important person. Not only Mr. Yen, but a large entourage also waited to greet us. Even a motorcar was placed at our disposable during our entire stay. Mr. Yen had engaged rooms for us at the Shanxi Hotel, so the manager of the hotel also embraced us. From the moment of our arrival, they relieved us of all responsibility as to our luggage, tickets, and so forth. All the details of our trip from there on were taken care of by our hospital host, who I might add also didn't speak a word of English.

Fortunately for us, Mr. Yen's Chinese secretary had a considerable Western education therefore was able to act as our interpreter. Upon entering the hotel lobby, they asked us to please give our Chinese names as well as our Western names for the register. Each of us had our cards, one side giving our Chinese name and address and the other side had the same printed in English. Calling cards when traveling in China were just as necessary, and even more useful, than a passport.

205

The hotel was managed under French management, the same as the railway. The menus were printed in French and the meals were fairly good for China if you excluded the coffee and shut your eyes to the swarms of flies.

Our host and accompanying friends escorted us upstairs to a private dining room that they had reserved for their foreign guests. They had an elegant banquet of food spread out on a table for twelve people. Following the use of Chinese custom, we all sat down to sip tea and exchanged greetings.

Miss Bullington and I did not mention the food we ate before in Taiyuanfu. We decided beforehand to prepare against emergencies by having a meal from our hampers before reaching our destination. This made it difficult to explain the situation when we they invited us to eat dinner. After a little explaining, the matter was straightened out and the dinner was postponed until the following day. Our friends stayed with us until almost ten o'clock.

Mr. Yen promised to call on us the following morning, around eleven o'clock, to take us around the city. I don't believe I'd ever slept in such an uncomfortable bed. Our pillows were filled with sand instead of feathers. A tired horse can sleep anywhere but I was physically exhausted having had only a little sleep the previous night, so despite the uncomfortable bed, we slept late until the following morning.

We went into the restroom to get ready because we were expecting breakfast to arrive, but to our surprise our host knocked at the door and without waiting for an answer, walked right in. We had to remember that when living in the Orient, the customs of the people were so different that anything could happen. We induced Mr. Yen to drink tea with us while we finished getting ready and ate our breakfast. Shortly thereafter, we left the hotel and began a tour of the city.

206

Like many of the other old northern Chinese cities, walls surrounded Taiyuanfu. The foreign hotel was situated outside the barrier. We drove through the narrow streets until we came upon a wide, long thoroughfare and arrived at a big market.

We entered through a large wide gate and passed many little shops, until finally reaching the important center courtyard.

It is famous for its lacquered chests in the innermost shops; we saw exquisite lacquered goods, rare curios, and ancient artifacts. The dealers from Shanghai and Peiping made regular trips into Taiyuanfu to pick up old valuable pieces and to find rare Ming or Sung curios. As we walked through the streets, we saw practically no other foreigners visiting the town and the town people considered us curiosities and were amused by the sight of us.

The following day, Mr. Yen picked us up and we drove out into the country to one of the most beautiful old temples I'd had ever seen in China. We were told that there were some bronzes there that were 4,000 years old. The pillars of the temple differed from any I have seen. Enormous gold lacquered dragons entwined the red- painted pillars. The effect of this, with the reflection of the broad noonday sun, illuminated the town. The courtyards of the temple had some fine old cedar trees, which were over 500 years. Under the trees in the courtyard temple ran a stream of crystal clear water, which flowed over some white rocks giving the appearance of an enchanted garden.

On our return to the city, Mr. Yen took us to his home. It was the first time I'd actually stayed for any length of time in a Chinese home, which led to the Western influence brought to bear on it. The general arrangement of a Chinese home differs from that of the Western world. All of the rooms open into one courtyard, but if the house is a pretentious one, there were many courtyards varying in size. During the summer months they placed a large sheet of grass matting above the courtyard to keep it protected from the elements.

We entered the outer door painted in a bright red, which contrasted beautifully with the dull grey cement wall. There were pots of flowers; pomegranate shrubs; oleanders; and wicker chairs, tables, and benches distributed in between the garden area. Our host asked us if he we would be interested in looking around the house and we accepted his invitation.

We walked through the living room, bedrooms, banquet hall, and a smaller dining room, which were all beautifully furnished. We saw old redwood Chinese beds, teakwood tables inlaid with mother-of-pearl old ivories, a beautiful lacquered chest, and boxes of camphor wood. The chests, all attractively embossed, came with Chinese locks.

Our invitation extended to the culinary department. The kitchen provided a modern Chinese stove, from which private delicious delicacies were produced. The Chinese people themselves have but two meals a day around ten in the morning and the next, between five to six in the evening. That evening, Mr. Yen invited several Chinese officials to a banquet in our honor. Miss Bullington and I used our small Chinese vocabulary to the best of our ability. We had a lovely time and learned a great deal about the area.

The morning of our departure, the chauffeur and car waited outside the door of the hotel to take us to the last 100 miles of our journey. We had a pleasant ride in a very comfortable car, which is a rare treat in China. We passed many old Ming tombs that dated back to the thirteenth and fourteenth centuries. Our friends from Yenching University, Dr. and Mrs. Learmonth, joined us before we left so they too had the benefit of Mr. Yen's kindness in transportation to our final destination, which was the valley of Yutacho.

Our traveling companions brought two servants from their house that took charge of our luggage. They traveled over 90 miles on an old rickety bus. At Fenchow, Mr. Yen's car dropped us off and took the Learmonths the last ten miles into the valley.

208

We arrived at Yutacho, crossed a stream, and were greeted by our new neighbors who invited us into their home. We took part in the cup that cheers, while our servants prepared our house and lit the fire to heat water for cooking purposes. We learned all the drinking water had to be carried from a mountain spring close by and every mouthful had to be boiled before it could be used in any way. Therefore, we hired a young Chinese boy whose chief work in life was to be a water carrier.

In the valley near our rental there were about 80 watermills, but only a few were still in operation. Each of these mills offered a charm of its own and was set along a fast-moving stream. Our rental house had one porch the entire length of the house, which served as a living room. We used another porch on another side of the house for our sleeping quarters. At the center of the large room, an old millstone still remained and served as a table for those meals. Most of the old mills had been converted into summerhouses. The ceilings were lofty with wooden beams that ran across the ceiling and the floors were made of flagstone.

The sound of rushing water from the stream that flowed by our door provided us with a free orchestra. The trees were mostly old stately elms about 80 feet high. The Chinese trees, named "scacia," are handsome leafy trees surrounding the area, mixed in with a few poplars and some old gnarled cedar trees hundreds of years old.

The valley was extremely fertile. I had never seen such crops— wheat, millet, corn, kaoliang, and cotton—and the fruits were luscious, including tomatoes, peaches, apples, and melons. The vines were happy with grapes or walnuts and other fruit trees laden with an abundance of God's sweetest treats. To the east, the mountains stood about 7,000 feet above sea level. The air was so fresh and cool, free from dust and delightfully bracing.

Fresh eggs and chickens cost us next to nothing. We bought eggs, 100 for 50 cents, and a good size chicken sufficient for four or five people for about twelve cents. Our neighbors, who had fruit and vegetable gardens, were constantly sending contributions of delicious young, sweet corn, tomatoes, melons, peaches, and other fruits.

We brought butter and milk in cans from the city cows in China, which were rarely seen and not used by the native Chinese people. Australian butter came into China in large quantities and, almost exclusively, foreign populations used it. Our cook made the bread and scones from the flour that was ground in an adjacent mill, the wheat being grown right behind my house.

We met one of our neighbors, Miss Disney, none other than a sister of Walt Disney, of Mickey Mouse fame. Ruth Flora Disney was a superintendent of the Chinese inland mission hospitals, and was nice, full of fun, and had a good sense of humor. What an excellent tonic a person with that kind of temperament is to a community, in any part of the world. Miss Disney's sense of ridiculous was always up for the most fun and we would go on the happiest adventures. We enjoyed spending time with her very much.

On either side of the valley, the mountainsides were terraced with the native's caves that they dug out from the mountains themselves. The opening through which one enters the dwelling is flush with the mountain. Inside there were mud walls, floors, and ceilings. Openings, oval or circular, were the only means by which air and sunlight passed into these rooms. A crude stove, usually made of mud bricks furnished the heat even in the coldest days in the winter when the temperature dropped to zero.

A large wide slab of stone constituted the family bed and had a sheepskin covering. The occupants lay crosswise, not lengthwise

210

as we do. In this way, six people are accommodated in one bed, usually the entire family of men, women, children, and babies. A clever device was brought out for winter only whereby the bed has a stovetop pipe beneath it. The pipe leads from the stove and carries hot air so that during the cold winter nights the natives slept in a heated bed at night.

We visited several native mountain families in the mud dwellings and they invited us inside. It was surprising that in the more prosperous cave dwelling homes we saw some thin pieces of furniture: old wooden trunks and old redwood cupboard end tables. Straw matting covered the floors and in winter they sealed up the windows with matting, but in summer everything was open to the world.

A queer little stovepipe jacks out above the terrace. This was their chimney and all summer long, tiny rings of smoke could be seen curling up from the hillside as the stoves offered the only means the natives had of cooking their food year round, as well as their heating in winter.

They were friendly people and welcomed foreigners. They even returned our call and brought us some little sesame cakes to show their good feeling. The only means of transportation into the valley of Yutacho was on mule. One travels with one's luggage in the panniers on either side of the mule, bedding provided by the only saddle. These sure-footed little animals climbed the mountain pass and crossed the stream at all times, day and night.

On one of our greatest expeditions, we used shanks mares on one full day's climb to over 5,000 feet. It was a fifteen-mile hike to the top and back, but we saw the glorious views of the mountaintops and plains below for miles and miles. We found a variety of wildflowers and other hardy specimens. We gathered multi-colored bouquets of flowers and grass, which we found growing and a little sequestered in the hollows thousands of feet up the mountain slopes.

211

On some of our rambles, we discovered pagodas and temples of ancient Sung and Tang dynasties, for Shanxi province posted as one of the greatest wealthiest of age in China. Fenchow had become a part of its wall and city gate, which is still standing, and that predates the Christian era some 3,000 years ago. We climbed every hill we could find. It was back to nature, making for a quiet and restful holiday filled with new interests.

One day we came across some old Manchu priests guarding the relics of the past at their mountain temple. They were the direct descendants of the royal family, Ch'ung, who conquered the Mongols in 1644 and established their own temples and palaces throughout the northern part of China. These priests only existed by the cultivation of the soil alone.

The valley of Yutacho is a veritable Garden of Eden, perhaps one of the most fertile valleys in the whole of China. It was a real privilege to visit such a beautiful area of China where the sun sets behind vast mountain stretches and only temple bells toll out their watches of the night. I found it so quiet and peaceful, and years later yearned to return.

Peiping, China: November 1935

In November 1935, it had been three and a half years since I left America for the Orient. In six months, I would complete my four-year contract. The board of the college wanted me to sign on for another four years. I agreed and requested a four-month leave of absence from my duties before I began my next contract. They added another two months for travel. My reappointment contract stated I would resume my duties as the Chief Physiotherapist for the period of July 15, 1936 to June 30, 1940.

I met a wonderful new friend, Mrs. Hayes, who had lived in the Far East for about twenty years. During these years she was a student of the Asian art and culture of the Orient. She was also an exceptionally fine mother of two daughters: Marion, age seventeen, and Janet, eleven.

212

It would be difficult to find two more delightful youngsters. They were usually appreciative of the beauties of nature and handcrafts, both ancient and modern, which we saw, and they were also delightfully spontaneous and refreshing in their enthusiasm and reactions.

On the morning of June 3, at 8:45 a.m., we left Peiping with a big send-off from our college friends, from both students and the faculty. Mrs. Hayes, her girls, and I left en route to America.

At noon we stepped aboard the S.S. Choju Maru, one of the steamers owned by the O.S.K. Lines that sailed between China and Japan by way of the Yellow Sea and the beautiful Inland Sea The Yellow Sea, like the English Channel, has a reputation of being more or less squally. On June 4, it did not belie its reputation, however, on the next day, the sea was not so rough. By morning of June 6, we had reached the bar of Jorje. On the account of the low tide, we went ashore in a tender, past Japanese customs, and soon we were on the ferry heading to Shimonoseki.

The Japanese women aboard the ferry were much entertained by the arrival of four Americans. They were of the peasant class, wearing a clean, pretty cotton native kimono, white cotton stockings, and the wooden sandals, known as *geitas*. The older woman still adópted a more elaborate Japanese style of hairdressing; the younger women had a much simpler mode.

A group of women sitting vice-a-versa were passing candy among themselves from neat little packages. One of the older women offered Mrs. Hayes' eleven-year-old, Janet, a piece. With a sense of awe and wonderment, the Chinese woman stroked the child's beautiful golden hair. The blue eyes and light hair of foreigners was a constant source of interest and bewilderment to the Oriental, in contrast to the black eyes and hair of their native people.

After reaching Shimonoseki, we still had about a four-hour train trip and a short ferry to reach our destination, which was the small island of Miyajima.

213

This island came into repute because of the famous Shinto temple that faces the bay. At high tide the water comes completely under the foundation of the temple. They built it in the seventeenth century on piles driven into the sand, similar to the foundation of Venice. The architecture was of a simple Shinto style; there were clusters of small temples on either side of the main one. Several feet out in the bay, and facing the temple in the famous red *torii*, was the gateway to the shrine, which had two uprights with cross pieces and stood 40 feet high on its foundation, entirely underwater.

We entered the temple and immediately took off our shoes. During the time we visited the temple, we noticed several pilgrims and worshipers praying. Their large hats distinguished the pilgrims, besides a knapsack strapped to their backs, and each carried a   tall staff. The worshipers knelt in front of the shrine and bowed their heads in prayer. At the same time, they clapped their hands twice, in order to call the attention of the gods. They repeated this frequently between prayers.

Mount Misen makes a remarkably beautiful background for the temple at about 2,000 feet high. At the summit there is a Shinto temple and torii. En route to the summit, we saw temples and several outlook platforms in the zigzag on a wooded path, which wound its way to the top. At the top, there was a grand view off the grey temple roofs, sea torii, and woods. We arrived at a little town with one narrow main street that was clean and well kept. Many gift shops with small Japanese hotels and restaurants lined the main thoroughfare.

The latter had its own little courtyard, which had a rocky garden with manicured shrubbery. It was watered from continuous spray, each courtyard having an individual pool. These gardens could be seen from the main street to the attractive opening of the door.

A flight of steps led to the Temple of the Thousand Mats they built in 1587. The mats and scrolls are inscribed in Japanese characters and hung on temple walls. Thousands of rice paddles stuck between the temple pillars, in which were the names of some worshipers who paid a considerable sum of money for the privilege of contributing a paddle.

An overnight train trip brought us to Kyoto, the city in Japan, which still retains a great deal of antiquity and ancient charm. The city of Kyoto lies in a bowl surrounded by wooded hills, which seems to be an intimate part of the city. Many small beautiful Shinto and Buddhist temples lie along the hillsides and streams flow from the hills, which run between the city and under bridges, some wide and long, and some narrow and short.

We spent a week in Kyoto at the home of one of the professors of Doshisha University, located about two and a half miles from the center of the city. We met some of Kyoto's distinguished leaders, both Japanese and foreigners.

Although Kyoto has many renowned temples, one being the Higashi Hongan-ji, known as the East Buddhist Temple, is one of the largest buildings in Japan. There were 96 huge pillars that support its great up-sweeping tiled roof. The former temple on the site was burned in 1879 and the present one was built by means of private contributions. Women who are unable to contribute either labor or money cut off their long black tresses to make ropes for hoisting immense pillars. Several of the human hair ropes were still preserved and could be seen under glass display in one of the corridors of the temple.

When we entered the main temple, hundreds of pilgrims were kneeling in front of the shrine. Buddhist priests were chanting before the bowed heads of the assembly. Straw mats covered the floor. The worshipers sat upon their legs in native fashion. The main portion of the temple seats around 1,000 worshippers.

215

Our guide told us that the farmers and peasants visited from the outlying districts to make pilgrimages, some only once in a lifetime.

We saw one of the pilgrimages. Mothers and grandmothers brought their offspring, while old, weary field workers who spent the greatest part of their working hours ploughing and in muddy swamps in the rice paddies, donned fresh, grey cotton kimonos. They traveled many miles in order to pay homage to the great Buddha and probably to do penance for a lifetime. The priests chanted the prayers as the twinkling of coins were evident—tossed into the nearest temple coffer by hand from each and every pilgrim. We crossed the city to the most beautiful temple, known as the Amida Buddha or the Kwonnon Buddha, which was situated on the southwestern slopes of the hill, from where the visitors can see the beautiful surroundings and great views of the city. The temple was known as Kiyomizu-dera.

They built it under both Shinto and Buddhist influence for the goddess of mercy. The vermilion torii was seen at the entrance of the Shinto temples as a symbol of sun and ancestor worship. The imposing torii of the seventeenth century guards the entrance of the temple, which were approached by a flight of stone steps on either side of which were two gigantic granite Korean lions.

At the top of the flight of steps stood a terrace with a large bronze figure of Amida Buddha; a picturesque old Campanile house bell made of bronze from 1620 AD. There was a penance pool at the entrance of the temple. Before entering, payment was required. Each man would strip, wearing a loincloth only, and stand in the pool while a stream of water from above fell upon his head and shoulders as his head was bowed in penance.

Kyoto boosts the Museum of Fine Arts in which exquisite pieces of furniture, especially lacquer inlay with ivory impressive stones, were housed.

Beautiful Japanese ornaments, scrolls, screen panels, paintings, and etchings were also on exhibit. There is a delicacy in form, color, and design about Japanese art, which I found enthralling and resonated with.

216

The old imperial palace in Kyoto stood in a large beautiful park that covered quite a large section and only a small section of it was open to the public—more beautiful inside and more unusual outside as Kyoto's castle. It belonged to the chief shogun, Mikado, who served directly under the Emperor. The capital moved to Tokyo in 1867, at which time the Mikado family no longer lived in the heavily fortressed and turreted castle.

The exquisitely decorated ceilings and gold leaf panel walls with their sliding doors, the polished lacquer floors, decorated, and dull golds with soft natural colorings, which harmonize so beautifully with a soft brown of the extensive, would work; all were designed with such similarity to the city. The lack of gaudiness is sad, satisfying, and peaceful.

One of our most interesting experiences in Kyoto was when we attended the Noh School of Classical Japanese involving music, dance, and drama. The theater was named Noh after a man named Zeami during the Muromachi period from 1333 to 1573. His work attracted the patronage of the government. The present actor, Congo, was the fifth of his generation to be in charge of the school. The art began in the fourteenth century together with Kyōgen. They performed in the old Noh theater where the actors' slow created movements conveyed to the audience a poetic language, in a monotonous tone.

The highlight of the performance was the old costumes from 1400 AD. They fortunately gave us box seats next to the imperial household. The play we saw dated back about 500 years and, by the kindness of our host, we were introduced to Congo, who played a leading role in the second of the three plays scheduled for that day. He graciously presented each of us with a portrait of himself and one of his old costumes.

217

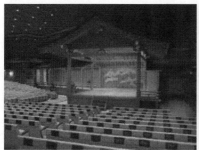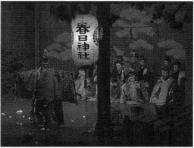

Noh School of Classical Japanese Theatre

Having been well informed about the play beforehand, we found no difficulty following the story. We were much impressed with the cadence and soft inflection of Congo's performers, especially in the singing parts. All of the actors' slow movements and gracefully executed timing created a marked precision. The story, a tragic one, was accompanied by three instruments: a flute-like instrument, a muffled drum, and one often used in Japan called a *samisen*, which is a cross between a guitar and a banjo with a square body, played with a large plectrum.

There were only male actors, of which some impersonated women. A cultured-looking group of people filled the audience and were most appreciative of their talents. Wooden slats had sectioned off the entire floor of the theater, some larger and some smaller, occupied by men and women who sat on rattan mats on the floor. A few boxes were positioned around a semi circular portion opposite to the stage slightly raised above the floor level, which provided the arrangement of the stage for the actors' entrances and exits. Their performance was true art in motion and was created right before our eyes.

218

We took an hour or two by rail from Kyoto to a little town of Omi-Hachiman. Dr.Willam Merrell Vories, an American, sometimes spoken of as the "Grenfell of Japan," had given 30 years of his life to a magnificent piece of work. He was gifted with an executive's ability and educated as an architect. He settled, and by his laborers, without financial help from any outside source, established a mission, playground, a tubercular sanitaria and an excellent grade school in the town named the Obayashi Children's House.

In order to finance his project, he obtained the rights to manufacture, sell, and distribute Mentholatum, which was an ointment and deep heating rub. He employed hundreds of young men and women in this enterprise. The employees were allowed one half-day for the pursuit of study in the schools. This practice had been established in order that the people may be able to get an education at the same time they earned their livelihood.

Dr. Vories married a Japanese lady, Makiko of rank about fifteen years before at the Meiji Kakuin University Chapel. At the time of the marriage, her family had disinherited her legally because of her marriage with in occidental. Before her marriage, Mrs. Vories had received a Western education and was a graduate of Bryn Mawr College. Her altruistic ideas blended with Dr. Vories, so they decided instead of having their own family, on account of racial difference, to devote their lives to building up a successful life of work in their community. In all respects the couple lived with the people, sharing in every way financially and in service, any community life.

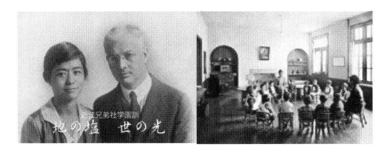

From Kyoto to Tokyo the railway carried people across some of the most beautiful country in the world—lakes, mountains, and glorious vistas of a shoreline, which reminded me of the French and Italian Riviera. The journey took about eight hours and the trains were clean, the service good, and meals were served in Japanese style.

Tokyo was very much like an up-to-date European city. It offered very little of the Oriental. The main streets are wide, clean, and exceedingly well kept and its office buildings and shops built in Western architecture, both inside and outside. They conducted business much the same way as in the Western world. Transportation by bus, car, or electric train service was excellent. There was little unemployment and very little, if any, evidence of poverty in any of the largest cities in Japan, although I had heard on good authority that the rural parts of Japan had considerable poverty.

A person took an electric train from Ueno station and in about three hours reached the beautiful Nikko. The little village was located about a quarter of a mile from the park. The visitor approached the famous old Japanese cedar walk that led to the red lacquer bridge with richly decorated five-story pagoda and an enormous bell.

The beautifully decorated temples, shrines, and mausoleums are reached on the other side of the stone steps surrounded by flowering shrubs and giant cedars. The temple at the top contains very old relics, gems, priest robes, jade, and frescoes.

Even more beautiful than that was the scenery at Lake Chūzenji in Nikko, which we reached by motorcar in three hours on a twisty road, with hairpin turns over 4,000 feet above sea level. The lake seen was completely surrounded by mountain ranges; the village had one of the largest copper mines in Japan.

220

We continued up the mountain to Lake Chūzenji. The clear magic crystal of the water, the mammoth cedars along the banks of the mountain enveloped the whole like a mantel of green and was truly enthralling. From an opening in the mountainside, hot sulfur springs bubbled and sprouted; bamboo pipes brought the steaming hot natural spring water to the Hotel Nanna, a well-kept Japanese secret hotel at which we spent the night.

Fortunately, an extremely kind Japanese man, Mr. Yen, formerly a student of Columbia University, who Mrs. Hayes had befriended, accompanied us. Without a Japanese-speaking companion, we would have fared rather badly at Yumoto, as not one member of the hotel spoke or understood English.

Many Japanese customs differ radically, even from those of oriental countries, such as the discarding of shoes at the entrance into any building, sitting, or sleeping on the floor, and the community baths. Our quarters for the night observed all of these customs and by persuasion and a little extra tip, Mrs. Hayes and I managed to wrangle about a half hour of the steaming hot tank. Before entering the community tank, each person bathes with soap and water and a small wooden square bucket for rinsing. We stepped into the tank, which was about twelve feet long by eight feet wide. Other inlets pouring in ice water balanced the continuous intake of natural mountain sulfur springs.

Upon returning to our rooms, we found three padded quilts to be used on the floor; the third provided covering. One medium-sized hard, round pillow was allotted to each person and neatly arranged on the floor of our sleeping rooms. They also provided a cotton kimono and a blue-padded fancy kimono for each of us.

A mirror on a stand about two or three feet high was our only piece of furniture and one of the two shelves built into the wall provided wardrobe space for our folded clothing. The experience of sleeping and eating on the floor level was more novel than comfortable to a Westerner.

221

Quite a number of the men in the audience wore Western clothes and a majority of the women wore attractive kimonos with a decorate *obi* and a number of older women still clung to the older more elaborate style of hairdressing. There were a good many geisha girls seated in boxes. They can be distinguished by the very elaborate hairdressing and flashy hair ornaments. Japanese women know the art of facial makeup and cosmetics and were the real beauty specialists of the world.

We experienced short intervals of fifteen minutes dispersed throughout the seven hours that the play lasted. People flocked into the foyer where they served refreshments; others carried small artistic double- and triple-decker locker boxes containing Japanese food. They manipulated their rice, salted dry, fresh seaweed, or pickles with the aid of chopsticks.

We visited St. Luke's Hospital and felt a most worthwhile experience, as it is very different than other hospitals I had seen. A modern day hospital is a place equipped with the most modern devices in the operating room, wards along with these essentials; this hospital also had a most unusual addition.

It stands as a monument to the ideas and ideals of Dr. Teusler who, 30 years ago, was a struggling medical missionary; this man had an idea of just such a hospital—one that has the comforts and atmosphere of someone's home. Every ward had its own vitaglass large circular sun porch and it's sitting room most artistically furnished and attractively arranged with a delightfully homey-like waiting room opened for the friends and relatives who came to visit their sick.

Rooms and meals for the friends and relatives were provided at it for even more moderate rates than those of a hotel, and also offered excellent cafeterias inside the hospital building. After spending two hours of rounds at the hospital, I remarked, "This hospital was not alone planned by architects and builders, doctors and nurses. It has the earmark in every detail of being planned by a person who loves and knows the needs of those who were suffering from physical, mental, and emotional elements."

The entire top floor had a dome of glass that was used as a solarium and kitchens had the latest devices in equipment. They had their own ice plant. The heating system was taken care of by oil burners and the tanks were fed from outside by an underground piping system. Within the building, even the Shinto type chapel was provided where either Eastern or Western religions rights may be observed.

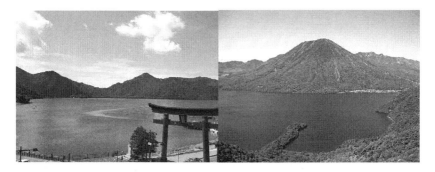

Looking out from Hotel Nanna Lake on Lake Lake Chūzenji in Nikoo, Japan (above) and 1935 Imperial Palace Entrance (below) Courtesy of the National Digital Collections

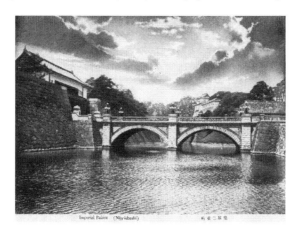

223

Our final journey was to meet Princess Kitashirakawa. Through the kindness of a friend, we were invited to the Imperial Shinjuku Palace to meet the present Emperor. When we arrived, we were customarily presented to her and graciously received. The princess was a widow, about 50 years of age. She wore a black net and lace Western style dress with a small black toque.

She was accompanied by her maiden-in-waiting and by her chief steward. We were escorted through the gardens with their long sleeping lawns, ponds having a large square stones and Buddhistic lamps placed at intervals around the banks. Picturesque fresh green shrubbery, clumps of purple irises, and banks of pink azaleas could be seen through a framework of gnarled and twisted cedars. Several hundred gardeners were constantly at work and palms were dredged at regular intervals to provide rich fertile soil for the flowerbeds and the view from the steps of the palace was particularly magnificent.

After two hours we paid our gracious princess farewell in order to catch a train out of the city. Before leaving, however, we heard, with much interest, more of the family's life of this charming lady from the person who so kindly made this interview possible—the story and life of Princess Kitashirshawa and her family, in addition to certain members of the Imperial Family.

This princess was not only the acknowledged daughter of the late imperial house but also the daughter of a geisha, a favorite concubine. Because of this, her sympathy and understanding with the people inspired her to vow that her two daughters should break away from their imperial heritage and marry men of their own choice. The princess accomplished this, but her only son, as the next heir to the throne, belonged to the country.

We were told an interesting story that was also connected with him. For a while her son was visiting in the United States and he fell in love with Matsudaira's daughter, whose father was the Japanese Consul in Washington during the time that the young member of the Japanese Imperial Family was visiting.

224

With much intrigue, and with the aid of the present Emperor, a match culminated in a royal wedding, but before the ceremony could take place, the bride to be, a commoner, had to be adopted into the Imperial Family.

After spending a few weeks in more or less intimate contact with the Japanese people, one appreciates many likable qualities. They were keen-minded, alert, fair in business dealings, courteous, and friendly to foreigners. Their cities were clean, well-kept, and the country was fully cultivated. Traveling was made easy and inexpensive. There were many public parks and gardens throughout the entire country.

Among the people, one sees a sense of earnest worship, not a perfunctory kneeling before the myriads of a shrine, but rather an innate sense of need for devotion and reverential attitude of the masses towards their temples and shrines. This typifies very different characteristics from the usual ones that the world associates with Japan today, such as the desire for unfair conquest, intrigue, and secret service, or the ruthless way they downtrodden Korean people and are now on their way to do the same in North China.

The unlikable qualities of Japan were not to be found in the Japanese people, but can be directly given to those in charge of the military system, who hold Japan's citizens at its merciless clutches. It is a military despotism that dominates Japan today—economically, educationally, and practically in every other way. This is the reason why the world in general distrusts the Japanese people and they were not held in greater esteem at the time.

As we stepped aboard the train at Tokyo, which took us on a 24-hour journey into Moji on the west coast, we were ready to embark on a little steamer. We hoped we would land there in about eight hours to Korea. We bid farewell to Japan with feelings of respect for all that had been preserved of the arts and handicrafts, for the perseverance that had mastered the industries of the occidental world, yet with the feeling of thankfulness to be free, unrestricted from the constant government surveillance which cramped the soul and the mind, and the freedom to speak one's thoughts, living one's life without having to bow before the tyrannical rule of military despotism.

225

Do you know the few lines that so graphically describe the king? "All among the yellow field the city stands, the walls keep watch, the gates lift up their heads, scorning the passing of the unguarded years, indifferent to affection or reproach, dead to remorse or help." By the time I reached Boston again, there would be just about two months until I set sail abroad again. I was eager to see my family and friends in America and see how the American Physical Therapy Association (APTA) was coming along since I was away. The time flew by and I was happy to be home again.

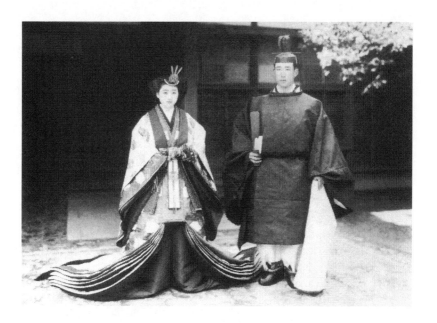

Imperial Prince and Princess Kitasirakawa's wedding day 1935

226

COMMITTEE ON THE HOSPITAL

December 9th, 1935.

Through an oversight the question of Miss McMillen's leave of absence was omitted in the Resolution presented to the members of the Hospital Committee at the meeting held on December 3rd.

The following resolution is therefore presented for your approval or disapproval:

RESOLVED   That the Committee on the Hospital recommend to the Acting Director the re-appointment of Miss Mary McMillan as Chief Physiotherapist for the period from July 15, 1936 to and including June 30, 1940, with the understanding that she be granted leave of absence for four months, and two months for travel, from July 15, 1936.

----------- *S. T. Wong*

	Approval	Disapproval
Dr. H. Loucks		
Dr. Maxwell		
Dr. Dieuaide		
Dr. Kronfeld		
Dr. I. C. Yuan		
Miss Whiteside		

Peiping University Medical College correspondence

Dr. S. T. Wang   December 23, 1938.

Director's Office

        T he following resolution re: reappointment of Miss Mary McMillan

as Chief Physiotherapist was passed by the Hospital Committee on December

3rd, 1938:
RESOLVED That the Committee on the Hospital recommend to the Acting Director
          the reappointment of Miss Mary McMillan as Chief Physiotherapist
          for the period from July 15, 1938 to and including June 30, 1940,
          with the understanding that she be granted leave of absence for
          four months, and two months for travel, from July 15, 1938.

        STW:K

January 2, 1936

Miss Mary McMillan
Peiping Union Medical College Hospital
Peiping

Dear Miss McMillan:

I have the honor to inform you that on recommendation of
the Committee on the Hospital you have been reappointed as
Chief Physiotherapist in the Hospital of the Peiping Union
Medical College for the period from July 15, 1936 through
June 30, 1940 with salary at the rate of US$3500 per annum.
You have also been granted leave of absence for six months
including travel time beginning July 15, 1936.

In all other respects the terms of this appointment are
the same as in your present appointment as outlined in
Miss M. K. Eggleston's letter to you of June 29, 1932. If
there are any material points relating to your appointment
which are not covered in our correspondence, kindly inform me
at once so that the official record may be complete.

If you agree to accept this appointment upon the terms
and conditions stated above, will you please sign and date
the acceptance at the foot of the enclosed carbon copy of this
letter and return it to me?

Sincerely yours,

J. Preston Maxwell
Acting Director

Superintendent of the Hospital

Date_____

I accept the foregoing
appointment upon the terms and
conditions outlined above.

Signature_____

February 10, 1936

Miss Mary McMillan,
Peiping Union Medical College,
Peiping.

Dear Miss McMillan:

Supplementing my letter of January 3, 1936 offering you reappointment as Chief Physiotherapist in the Hospital, I wish to inform you that on recommendation of the Committee on the Hospital the leave of absence for six months including travel time beginning July 15, 1936, has been extended for two months to provide a total of eight months leave of absence including travel time, with the understanding that you will return to duty not later than March 1, 1937.

In all other respects the terms of the appointment offered you are the same as outlined in my letter of January 3, 1936.

If you agree to accept this appointment upon the terms and conditions stated in my letter of January 3, 1936 supplemented by this present letter, will you please sign and date the acceptance at the foot of the enclosed carbon copy of this letter and return it to me?

Sincerely yours,

J. Preston Maxwell
Acting Director

Superintendent of the Hospital   Date Feb. 11, 1936

I accept the foregoing appointment upon the terms and conditions outlined above and in the letter of January 3, 1936.

Signature _____

The Battle of Peiping: July 1937

During this period, I was on leave in America and became worried that the Shanghai International Settlement was the only politically neutral territory in east China. It was also one of the few places in the world that did not require a passport or a visa for entry, making it among the last refugee countries for European.

I returned to my duties at PUMC on July 15, 1936, and all went along as normal for about a year until the Japanese began to put more and more pressure on China to take over their power. We were not really worried that Japan would take over, but we still walked on eggshells not knowing what would happen

Jews were fleeing the Holocaust. Arriving first by sea and later on the Trans-Siberian Railway, the number of Jewish refugees in Shanghai reached almost 20,000.

These Jews, arriving from Germany, Austria, and Poland, lived throughout the city, both inside and outside the International Settlement. After 1943, they were forced to relocate to the Hongkou District, a ghetto established for stateless Jews. There were so many big changes happening around the world, and much uncertainty as to how it would affect our profession and my return to China.

At this same time, the Chinese magnificently held to their end of the agreement and were patient beyond measure, but insisted upon defending their country against Japan. There was a last chance for reconciliation, but neither side would give in and the citizens were proud to stand by them because we believed the Chinese shouldn't give in.

It surprised us to learn the Japanese were up to their tricks again since they'd agreed to a truce with China in 1922. On July 7, they crossed the border at Fengtai and attacked the walled city of Wanping. The Chinese fought back and the Japanese ordered the city to be shelled on July 9. The fighting continued and a huge battle broke out at Langfang on July 25, and ended bitterly two days later.

231

In 1937, I was reassured the APTA continued to grow as a nationwide organization. They sustained and maintained a professional and scientific standard for those engaged in physical therapy; the second thing was to propose the science of physical therapy. Also, they had a purpose to help in the establishment of educational standards and within scientific research in physical therapy. They also worked with people in the medical field. They provided information for those interested in physical therapy and created a central registry, which was made available to the medical profession.

Physical therapy physicians had achieved recognition as a medical specialty. In an effort to further distinguish themselves from physiotherapists and in order to gain respect within the medical profession, physical therapy physicians began to call themselves "physiatrists."

On July 28, 1937, a report informed us that the Japanese recaptured Langfang. At about 8:30 p.m., the firing began and within twelve hours the Chinese recaptured the most important three areas that had been capped red by the Japanese. The cities were Tientsin, Fengtai, and Lungchow, which were located just outside Peiping.

Fengtai is a vital spot to the north and south of R.R. Junction, so that meant not only a great moral victory made for the Chinese, but also one of the most strategic centers in North China was back in the hands of the Chinese. Our Generalissimo arrived by plane early that morning in Paotin, the new capital of the Hopi province and the troops poured into the south.

I shall never forget the fear, anxiety, and terror of that morning. I awoke around 5:00 a.m. on July 28 to the popping of guns. The gunfire lasted for several hours and then the roar of airplanes. flying close to the ground that seemed to almost touch the house roofs. Several of our medical students picked up sheets of paper dropped from the planes.

232

Written on the sheets were Chinese characters that read, "Much respected old people of China, after the insults from your young people of China following the Lukuchinao incident, we, the Japanese, who were so insulted and so troubled by this affair, have come with very big guns. You must not be alarmed, dear old people of China, you must trust us."

There was no such thing as lying in bed under these circumstances so I puttered around a little in my garden trimming, watering, and cutting for an hour or two to keep my mind off the impending danger. Around 8:00 a.m., an armed guard from the American Embassy came to escort me over to my safety zone, which happened to be at PUMC. I assured him I had no fear and he better escort some foreigners who might need his help.

The servants who attended my house were frightened because an American flag hung at my door. All my Chinese neighbors—men, women and children—walked out in the streets, while the airplanes kept buzzing and the roar of cannon seemed to get closer. The Chinese Army had piled thousands of sandbags up through the street corners connecting with the main highways. Fortunately, the police on duty knew me well, as they were not allowing anyone to pass, but thankfully, I got through. Some people at PUMC were not so fortunate. The police detained them, and it took over two hours to walk the fifteen-minute journey.

After I deposited my worldly goods in my office, at least some of them, I made myself busy. I had no other clothes except those I stood in and goodness knows how long I would be a prisoner at the college. Our dear Dean of Women came around to tell me that they assigned me a room and food would be provided so long as the supply would hold out.

I dismissed the members of my staff, professional and otherwise, according to instructions and kept only one assistant who lived outside the walls, so he couldn't get home in any case. I also kept one attendant who cared for hospital cases only, and no outpatients. This was by far our larger group and the hospital patients who were taken to and from the wards.

233

In the midst of fear, one must move forward as if everything is going to be okay, so we decided to continue working as normal and get some much-needed things done. I managed to invite one of our painters in the hospital who had a good deal of leftover paint to give the woodwork a first coat of paint.

We lived through the first day of occupation and none of us had any idea what the future held and we were afraid of considering one of the conditions in the Japanese ultimatum yesterday. They threatened that by twelve o'clock; noon that day, all the Chinese troops within the city should be withdrawn or Peiping would be shelled. It seemed as if our obstreperous friends might have to face their first disappointment thus far because Peiping was not shelled and the retaking of Fengtai was the grandest news we could get.

The foreigners here were so proud of any Chinese gain. We were afraid that parlays between Chinese and Japanese generals in Tientsin didn't sound too hopeful for China. Now that action had taken place with the backing of the South and General Chiang Kai-shek, new hope sprung up.

The following day at noon, while I was eating lunch, our Chinese staff members expressed the spirit resistance among the younger, more educated people and the fire with which they talked about, had been true all over China that day. Many of our young people had given up the idea of vacation or going to study abroad, and signed up for our emergency medical corps, clamoring to volunteer for the army and the Red Cross.

I could hardly bear to think of the sacrifice of life that this struggle means to the people of this country; of course one must see that from both sides. I was overwhelmingly glad that the Chinese had not submitted to merely handover any more of their country. They were willing to fight, and even die to keep their country and freedom from the Japanese.

234

Peiping, China: August 2, 1937

Since Japan threatened China on July 28, and the trains stopped running in Peiping, meaning we had no communication with the outside world except through the navy military station by radio for over a week while the fighting roared on.

On July 31, I sent my family a telegram to let them know the news of the impending war and that I was okay. This was the only means of communication with the outside world. The city had been closed off to the rest of the world and no one knew what was going on. It was a time of fear and uncertainty.

All of the city gates remained closed so no food supplies could enter the city. We had no vegetables, no rice, no meat, and no fish. During this time we had to subsist on canned goods besides flour and rice. Most foreigners stayed within their own legations. The fear of uncertainty as to what was going to happen became unbearable to many.

In the midst of the tension, several hundred Americans took refuge at the Embassy and set up camp on some of the most beautiful lawns outside the American legation for protection. Tents pitched five deep and tent poles were well utilized with baby's diapers. I went over to the American legation to see my former housemate, who was now established in a small apartment all to herself in one of the houses where the Embassy staff secretaries were. The mess hall of the Embassy guard had been turned into a community dining room, rich and poor alike, including American born Chinese plus a few stray tourists filed inside, side by side eating good American food just as it was served to the men in the barracks: meat, biscuits with gravy, and canned vegetables.

One family came in with eight children, father, mother, their amah, and a goat. It's clear why they brought the goat, as the children cannot survive without the milk. I believe the father was an American missionary from outside the city.

235

The American minister had gone to Nanjing, but the minister's wife was active in relief work. She turned over the lower floor of their home, ballroom, drawing, and dining rooms as dormitories for United States citizens.

We were okay until the morning of July 29, as the threat of dropping bombs on us continued. It was the risk of poisonous gases spraying over us this morning that was too much for the Chinese Army men to defend their country. They did not have adequate munitions or implements of warfare.

From my bed of safety in the hospital all night long, I heard the *pop, pop, pop* of guns early in the morning and a message from central government ordering the Chinese troops out of the city in order to prevent the hazard of gas bombs falling early that morning. We all felt it was a tragic situation. The Japanese walked in at about 11:00 a.m. with a new pro-Japanese mayor; his wife was Japanese and they took over. I prayed God would help the northern Chinese. I still had faith in the general and that he would save both the south and the interior given the time to prepare. July 29 was a very sad day for the north.

On August 3, the city of Peiping began to struggle drastically because there was no sewage except for a few houses rented by foreigners. We had no way of disposing of the garbage inside the city walls. The street corners became piled with city refuse and the smell overwhelmed the city. The volunteer organizations focused on taking care of the wounded and it was exceedingly difficult, even under the Red Cross, to get a pass to go out and return. Only one pass had been granted by the Japanese for seven Red Cross trucks to go out daily, manned by a volunteer corps of doctors and nurses close by from PUMC.

It is a blessing that space had been assigned to take care of all the wounded. We had a limited number of the worst cases in the hospital because it was an adequately kept institution. Besides the hospital cases, a great number of dressing changes for the wounded were performed in our outpatient department each day.

236

The little Chinese nurses for several weeks had been given their afternoon off to make hospital slings and other women's organizations were making bed jackets. As of August 4, the city was still shut off from the rest of the world. There were no trains, telegrams, telephones, or any communication. Japanese soldiers guarded the whole city but the main entrance to the Legation Quarter was not only heavily guarded by them but also blocked by barbed wire fences.

One of my nurses in the physical therapy department had a wife and five children in Tungchow, only about eighteen miles from Peiping, and he had no idea for a whole week whether they were dead or alive. He felt relieved to hear his family was still alive even though the area had been hit by heavy warfare.

The head college health physician and the head of the purchasing department returned from Peitinho ten days before and could get no farther than Tientsin; for days no one knew if they were alive until we finally heard they had safely arrived. The fighting continued to take place in Tianjin, but the Chinese finally retreated, and on August 8, the Japanese forces captured Peiping. On this morning, papers shared rather alarming news— apparently Russia had been making promises of a system of assistance of men and ammunition to China. The future looked bleak as, from this day forward, we were now living each day in a hot bath with the Japanese.

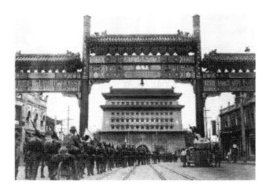

The Battle of Pieping July 1937

Peiping, China: 1938-1940

My contract with Rockefeller and PUMC would end in June 1940 and they were already asking me to stay on for another term. Even under the stress and fear of the Japanese invasion, I was seriously considering it. I had fallen in love with China—it's people, my home, dogs, and friends. It would be very difficult to leave, but I also missed my family and friends in America.

I decided to wait to answer them until I returned from my long awaited vacation. I received a five-month furlough. My sister Katherine would travel by boat to Peiping, China for the first leg of our journey. She spent the first few weeks with me in my home and I gave her a tour of where I worked. I wanted to share every detail about how much I had come to love China and its people.

We also traveled to the Japanese shrines first stopping at the Shrine Office which covers 551 tsubo, an area at the Shinto Shrine that offers a viewing of long neck vases called a *tsubo*, or a vase made of clay, and walked through the Choyo-kaku, the "Hall of Morning Light," which has an alter reached by a flight of stone steps. At the back of the museum lay a *Koyo-en*, that is, a sacred secluded garden filled with enchanting trees and foliage. We stood and gazed at the Ryūzu Falls, Kirifuri Falls, and Kegon Falls in Nikko that tumbled over rocks, foaming and roaring down the mountain. We visited Lake Chūzenji, a twenty-mile lake famed for its beauty. It is known as the Sachi-no-Umi, the "Lake of the Fortunate." I also took her to the Great Wall of China, which I had seen before, but my second visit was no less inspiring.

Kay was a schoolteacher and would have many wonderful adventures and photos to share with her class when she returned to America. We departed Kobe, Japan on August 7, 1940, on the boat, Hie Maru, and arrived in Seattle, Washington, on August 22[ns] We took a train back to Boston and it was nice to see and spend time with my family and friends again.

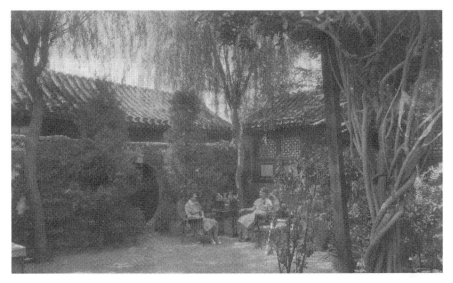

Garden photo of Mary McMillan and her sister, Catherine

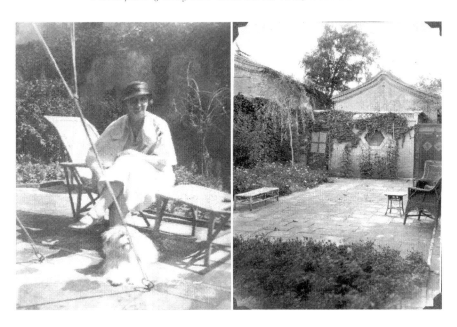

Relaxing in her gardens in Peiping, China

My Return to Peiping, China: 1941

After much communication with the Rockefeller Foundation and PUMC, I decided to return to China for another short contract to train and wrap up my work there. Even though there was still the threat of the Japanese, I believed all would be well and I would be safe. Why had I decided to stay? I can only say there was still more work to be done and I was inspired to serve the wonderful people of China.

I was sad, but also excited that physical therapy in America had ignited for a second time on June 1, 1941 and women signed up for emergency training courses for the World War II. Times had changed since 1918; instead of them being called reconstruction aides, they were now titled physical therapists. They trained to assist soldiers and possibly experience combat.

The profession had experienced many technological developments and the United States Army Medical Department came up with a strategy as to how they would rehabilitate the wounded soldiers—to include physical retraining, vocational rehabilitation, and psychological support.

When soldiers returned home, it was now possible for physical therapy to be practiced at their homes. The practitioners assisted in treatments like amputations, burns, cold injuries, wounds, fractures, and nerve and spinal cord injuries.

Drastic changes in the medical management of war wounds with penicillin and sulfa drugs, and improvements in surgical techniques, led to increasing numbers of individuals returning to the United States with disabling war wounds.

I jumped back into my work right away when I returned to PUMC. There was still the threat of the Japanese but I kept busy so I didn't have to worry. On July 5, 1941, I attended a luncheon at the American Club, which had not been held for a couple of years due to the fighting between China and Japan, but I still managed to celebrate it that year. I celebrated in several ways from noon until midnight, with a spot of work sandwiched in between, as we did not have a holiday on the 4th, even if we worked in an American institution.

240

I was invited to a swimming party luncheon outside the American Embassy pool. I took my bathing suit along but, having suffered with neuritis for over a week, decided against it. My friend Ann was the only person under the awning until lunch was served. I took a leisurely luncheon, and got back to the hospital around 3:00 p.m.

At about 6:00 p.m., I left the hospital and paid my respects to the acting Chief of the Embassy, which is a custom, and had become a tradition in Peiping by all American citizens. At 7:30 p.m., I left with the three ladies and nine gentlemen to have dinner out of doors at the lovely Peiping Palace. I found toast and soda water, which is a much better choice for a lady who was recovering from a severe case of acute neuritis.

In the evening under the moonlight, we danced over sculptured rock gardens surrounded by myriads of red lanterns, a white marble camelback bridge, beautiful trees, and Ginkgo growing abound beautiful gaily-painted balconies. Small red and black lacquer tables were strewn around the grounds. One long table with vegetable salads, chicken, rice, and other delicacies were laid out, and two cooks with high tall white caps straight over the open fires cooking and serving shaved strips of meat and sausages that they tucked inside a little hot dinner roll.

The day had been a scorcher, almost 100 degrees indoors, but turned out to be quite cool and pleasant. Following supper, fireworks were set up on the grounds. I was fortunate enough to be invited to go home in one of the Embassy cars, as it would take about 40 minutes by rickshaw and only ten minutes by car. The setting was so beautiful that it will remain in my mind as one of the most outstanding picturesque evenings in Peiping. I had not attended anything out of doors quite like it for years.

The following week, a doctor gave me a very thorough run of neurological tests and x-rays, and seemed to think I was deficient in vitamin B. Every day I had a vitamin B injection and was also taking six tablets, so all of my pain was gone. I was advised to take some time off to rest and recuperate.

241

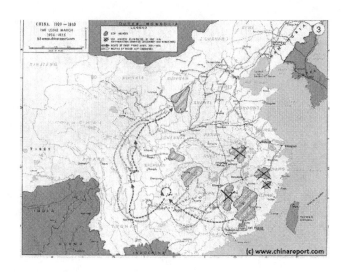

1930's China Map (above) and Sightseeing Map (below)

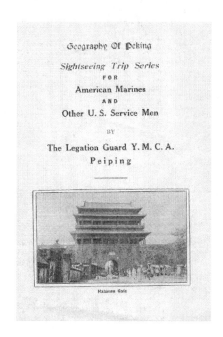

Tsingtao, China: Shandong Province and Edgewater Mansions Hotel

On July 13, 1941 I took a 24-hour journey by rail to the Shantung coast to a place called Tsingtao after going to the police and military bases to get all the necessary paperwork and photos. Since the Japanese occupation, one realized how easy it was to travel in America. It took a couple of days for me to take what was a normal two and a half hour trip. When one traveled in China during this time, one had to present three photos to each bureau to have papers filled out both from police and military headquarters before one could board a train.

I had looked forward to a change of scenery and routine. To be able to let down my hair for a few weeks and get some must needed rest after all the sleepless nights I had experienced the last year. I was dismayed when I was squashed into a compartment sleeper with a Japanese gentleman, his wife, and two children. From tea until sleeping time I had to deal with all of them, but fortunately, by bedtime, the family had moved to another compartment. It was cold but I was relieved when the family departed at the next stop.

I reached the town in 24 hours on July 14 to start my vacation. My young teaching student met me at the train and after some deliberation we drove three miles to the Edgewater Mansions Hotel. As the name implies, the hotel is right at the water's edge overlooking Tsingtao, which was part of the mighty Pacific Ocean. The building stood above a crescent-shaped beach. Woods, mountains, trees—especially pines—all around the coastline. The view reminded me very much of the pine trees in the states and made me mighty home sick. They built the luxurious hotel as a German showpiece in honor of the social events surrounding the coronation of King George VI.

They designed the hotel along modernistic lines from the outside. I thought the rooms exceptionally nice, large each having a small balcony overlooking the sea and a private bathroom. There was a stonewall enclosure, making a fine place for bathing. Every day I took swimming lessons. The cost was absurdly reasonable and it gave me something constructive to do instead of just lying around.

There were few foreigners in the hotel, mostly Japanese, so I spent much of my time alone.

My young Chinese student visited me every day in the afternoon and we enjoyed our many walks together. I knew him and his wife very well in Peiping a few years ago. I was happy to hear about all he had learned and what he had been doing at Shandong University. I walked every day even though my red face and arms hurt and were finally taking on a tan. I felt splendid and enjoyed my vacation immensely and it was worth the 24-hour train trip. I hoped the following summer I would be with my family in America, for I felt all the work done building PUMC hospital's physiotherapy program had been accomplished.

On July 21, during one of the most beautiful summers I have ever known, I took a delightfully pleasant stroll. I walked several miles from one coast to the next and unexpectedly ran into a man knew in Peiping from several years ago. It was Dr. Shields, the dean of the medical school, Cheeloo University. I went with him and called upon his wife, who promised to spend the day with me on the following Wednesday. Luckily for them, the doctor and his wife planned to leave next week to return to America.

The following day I had lunch at the United States Consulate by invitation of Paul Mira, head of the consulate office, who we used very much in the East. Every day was a wonderful and relaxing adventure. Each day and night as I laid on my bed, I had a splendid view of the bay, the red tile roofs, and cream-colored houses inserted among pine trees along the coast. It made me think of the French and Italian Riviera, with a clear blue sky and rocky ledges immersed between colors for several miles. And the sunset view from the dining room was a majestic site.

I was in no hurry to return to Peiping and the hospital, but my vacation was at an end, and it was time to return, although not for very long, as very soon I would finishing up my contract and sailing for a finally journey back to my true home: America.

244

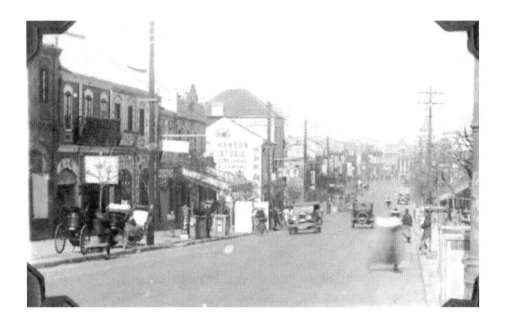

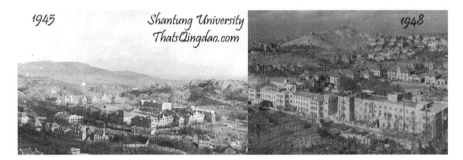

Cheeloo University

5021

2272 TSINGTAO 1202 12 9 40M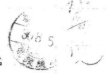

HOUGHTON ROCKEFELLER HOSPITAL PEKING

ARRIVE TUESDAY NIGHT PLEASE ADVISE MY HOUSE ~~MACMILLAN~~

MACMILLAN

Telegram notifying arrival to new house in Peking

CONFIRMATION OF CABLEGRAM

FROM

PEIPING UNION MEDICAL COLLEGE

PEIPING, CHINA

CODES:
GENTLEY'S
WESTERN UNION
MISSIONS

CABLE ADDRESS:
MEDICAL PEIPING

CABLEGRAM NO.

CODE USED

TO   LC   CHIMEDBORD   NEWYORK

November 25, 1940   19

DE WORD	TRANSLATION
	APPROVE MCMILLAN OUTGOING

CONFIRMATION OF CABLEGRAM

FROM

PEIPING UNION MEDICAL COLLEGE

PEIPING, CHINA

CODES:
BENTLEY'S
WESTERN UNION
MISSIONS

CABLE ADDRESS
"MEDICAL PEIPING"

CABLEGRAM NO.

CODE USED

V/YYY

CEIVED FROM: CHIMEDBORD   NEWYORK

Received on   November 24, 1940   19

DE WORD   TRANSLATION

DLT   MEDICAL   PEIPING

HOUGHTON CABLE EIGHTEENTH REFERRED ALL WOMEN BUT RESPONSIBILITY

DECISION RESTS WITH PARTIES IMMEDIATELY CONCERNED MCMILLAN VISA

SHOWS WASHINGTON NOT URGING EVACUATION ESSENTIAL PERSONS MCMILL

PREPARED SAIL DECEMBER SIXTH BUT ASKS YOUR APPROVAL

                                              LOBENSTINE

CONFIRMATION OF CABLEGRAM

FROM

PEIPING UNION MEDICAL COLLEGE

PEIPING, CHINA

CABLE ADDRESS "MEDICAL PEIPING"

CABLEGRAM NO.

CODE USED

CODES BENTLEY'S WESTERN UNION MISSIONS

711991

EIVED FROM: CHIMEDBORD NEWYORK

November 9th, 1940 19

DE WORD	TRANSLATION (Cable dated November 8, 19
	NLT MEDICAL PEIPING HOUGHTON ELECTION STRONG ENDORSEMENT PRESIDENTS FOREIGN POLICY STOP GOVERNMENT EVACUATION ADVICE PRECAUTIONARY MEASURE REDUCTION HAZARDS MCMILLAN VISA GRANTED LOBENSTINE

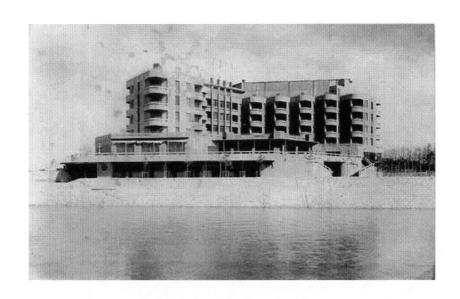

Edgewater Mansions Hotel (above) and

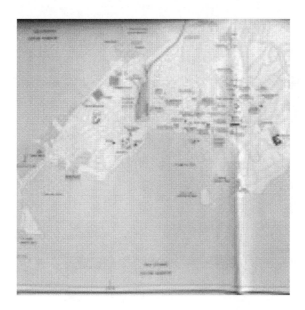

The city of Tsingtao

Tsingtao 1948-49

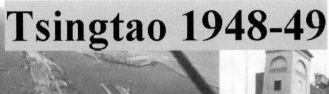

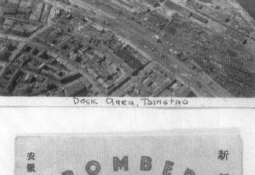

Dock Area, Tsingtao

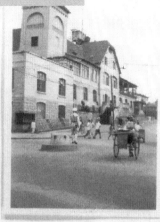

Tsingtao Scenes 1948

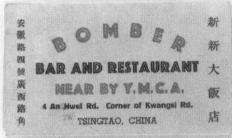

安徽路四號廣西路角

BOMBER
BAR AND RESTAURANT
NEAR BY Y.M.C.A.
4 An Hwei Rd. Corner of Kwangsi Rd.
TSINGTAO, CHINA

新新大飯店

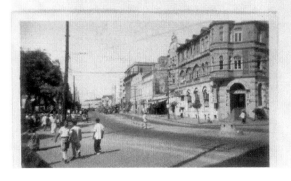

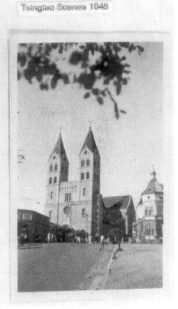

The city of Tsingtao

13

I SHOULD HAVE SEEN
THE SIGNS

October 27, 1941

I returned to my work at PUMC feeling much better and ready to fight another day. If I had been a fortune-teller and listened to my gut instincts, I should have returned to America during my time off instead of going to the seaside—but a McMillan's word is true blue and I had agreed to come back to the college to finish out my contract. The physiotherapy work went on as usual but not without the apprehension of unrest and uncertainty of what would happen with the Japanese.

It became evident after a couple months there was no time to waste and I needed to somehow find a way to get back to America, contract or no contract. Dr. Hart Houghton requested that we few "women folk" return to the States as soon as possible. He believed it would be difficult to carry on duties because of the anxiety about the occupation.

The college mostly had a native staff working and had been asked to endeavor and keep going as long as possible. The freezing of the funds for charitable and educational institutions would be a deathblow to all existing United States missions that were now functioning in China. We had to follow the same course as Korea did a long time ago. There was no need for me to comment on my feelings, as sometimes it does no good when you have no control as to what will happen.

The United States Consulate told the Americans at the hospital that there was no possible chance to travel before December but there could be a chance here or there, so to be ready for an eleventh hour notice. In any case, my name for a booking was already on the cook's passenger's list on the first boat out. I cabled to my family to let them know when and if anything was definite. The shipping attendant told me we might have to go to Manila and wait there for further booking. I prayed I'd reach Boston for Christmas, but the prospect looked bleak.

To share that I was concerned about the following events and sad to suddenly leave all my Chinese friends with whom I came to like so well, cared for, and was so happy to work with would be hard to write off. The crisis of uncertainty and panic left me no time to

Medical staff at Peking Union Medical College, China

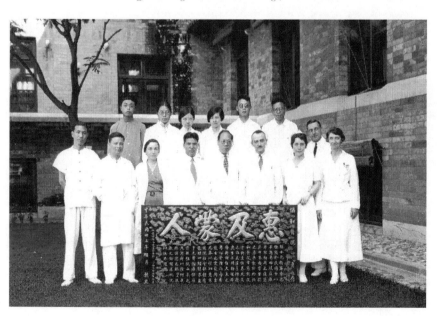

Mary McMillan at far right of the group

say proper goodbyes or offer my well wishes to anyone. I had to leave, and quickly.

I packed one small steamer trunk and a suitcase to travel with me. I prepared and hoped to be fortunate to take my personal effects but was perfectly resigned not to. I felt in a pinch, I could travel with my suitcase only and make do. One never knew what calamities could come before we left in December.

The hospital staff continued its work and the college choir decided to perform our annual symphony and choral concert. We had a full house on both evenings and the concert inspired many who needed some encouragement.

On November 2, 1941, one professor was booked to depart on the President Coolidge in a few days. I asked him to mail a letter to my family for me from the West Coast. It was a letter I'd written when on vacation—resting and being healed by the sun and sea breezes, restored in mind body and spirit. I wanted to reassure them that after my vacation, I was no longer concerned about my health. I told them that nothing, not even the Pacific Ocean and all the seven seas, could separate them from my love and spirit, and that I believed by the grace of God, we would be together soon.

After spending almost ten years in China, the day to leave finally arrived. I was strongly urged again to leave the country as soon as possible because of the possible eminence of a Japanese war. It is not that I had not tried; I had booked myself on several ships, but they had cancelled all those ships.

On November 14, 1941, I booked another passage with the Cook & Company on a boat for Peiping to Hong Kong to San Francisco on the S.S. San Francisco. If luck was on my side, I would be home in time for Christmas.

I took the train to Tientsin, spent two days at the Astor House Hotel, then boarded a steamer to Hong Kong via Shanghai, where

255

I spent over a week at the Palace Hotel trying to figure out what to do next as no boats were leaving for America.

By courtesy of the United States government, on December 5, 1941, some of my colleagues and I had been granted permission to travel from Shanghai to Manila, the Philippines, with the Shanghai Marines on a United States chartered steam ship, as no other vessels were available.

They took us from Manila to Baguio but when we arrived, the steamship office informed us that we would not be able sail from Manila before December 20. Therefore we traveled as a group up north about 150 miles into the hill town of Baguio to wait until the ship would be ready.

On the late morning of December 8, 1941 at 8:00 a.m., the seventh day in the Western Hemisphere, while breakfasting at the Pine Hotel in Baguio, the Philippines, we heard the announcement that was to electrify the world. They announced that the Japanese had attacked Pearl Harbor: "We are now in the midst of a war, not for conquest, not for vengeance, but for a world in which this nation, and all that this nation represents, will be safe for our children. We expect to eliminate the danger from Japan. So we are going to win the war and we are going to win the peace that follows. And in the difficult hours of this day—through dark days that may be yet to come—we will know that the vast majority of the members of the human race are on our side. Many of them are fighting with us. All of them are praying for us. But, in representing our cause, we represent theirs as well—our hope and their hope for liberty under God."

We sat in shock as President Roosevelt's voice was broadcasted on the United States special radio message from Washington, followed up by playing the "Star-Spangled Banner." Our country's national anthem took on a very vital significance; our hearts responded with thankfulness that at least we were on American territory at such a time—and the American President promised that help was forthcoming,

256

which soothed our anxiety. He asked that all people take heart. The Americans and Filipinos in Manila trusted his statement and truly believed America would prevail and win the war quickly.

My friends and I noticed the Quezon Cabinet had been sitting at the next table at the hotel and a look of terror spread over their faces. President Quezon and his cabinet immediately left Baguio in his private plane for Manila upon hearing the news of Pearl Harbor. The Japanese had been planning an attack on the Philippines for a long time. For years they had placed high-ranking officers in disguise as laborers and tradesman in all the key towns. The people were misled by the kindness of the Japanese spies and became their friends. There were rumors for years that an invasion was going to

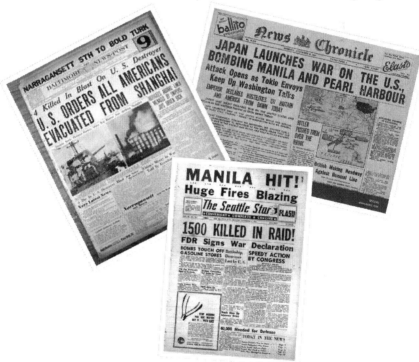

Newspaper headlines of the invasion on Pearl Harbor and Manila where the Japanese soldiers captured Mary McMillan and other detainees

happen, but no one knew when. Japanese incursions into China began as early as 1931, shortly after the Mukden Incident, which was a military operation that was a pretext to the invasion.

The following six years saw several smaller incursions, both military and political. In Asia, the Second Sino-Japanese War began with the full-scale Japanese invasion of China in 1937. Two years later, World War II began when Germany invaded Poland. The conflicts merged in 1941 when the United States entered the war following the Japanese attack on Pearl Harbor, Hawaii.

That same morning, native Filipinos and Igorots, who lived in the hills near Baguio, had brought in great quantities of tropical fruits red and yellow, bananas, luscious pineapple, and also crisp fresh green vegetables in abundance to sell that morning. Many natives also brought their handcrafts to the large open market in town. It was as if a thunderbolt had struck the place and the people's faces fell distraught and showed open consternation at the astounding war news.

Between nine and ten o'clock, air sirens began screeching and we rushed around the market trying to figure out what to do next. We listened to pitiful tales from the eager women who told us how they depended entirely upon making a living from the sale of their handicrafts to the white people, a beautiful assortment of which were on display.

A few Americans, and other white people with whom we talked to in small shops and in town, could not grasp that we were at war. We heard the air sirens screeching at close shot and were dizzy with fright. Yet we, as individuals, were all part of it, just as much as the United States soldiers stationed in our far-flung Army posts. It was difficult to orient all the mixed feelings we all felt as we knew in air bombing, there were no discrimination—soldiers and civilians alike share the same fate of becoming victims.

We walked outside, looked up at the sky, and saw Japanese war planes dropping bombs and explosions. One bomb dropped on the United States Army post gate, Camp John Hay, before noon of the same day. The wounded and the dying were being brought to the local hospital from Camp John Hay, so my friends and I immediately volunteered and did what we could to help.

258

Japanese forces broke the stronghold the Allied nationals held in the Pacific. By the afternoon, the Japanese attacked the main United States Air Base at Clark Field, and on December 9, 1941, the second day after hearing of Pearl Harbor during the first Japanese attacks, it was the earliest we could persuade the Filipino motorcar drivers to take us the 155-mile drive from the hills of Baguio to the city of Manila.

Before starting the journey, they told us it was necessary to obtain a military pass. Fortunately, one of our friends had met the Adjutant of Camp John Hay who kindly stamped our identifications with the army seal of General MacArthur, which listed us as Red Cross workers. The Japanese police patrolled all the roads and they often stopped us along our journey, but fortunately we passed our examination each time. Within a few miles of Manila, air raid sirens shrieked, and then we heard more booms in the air.

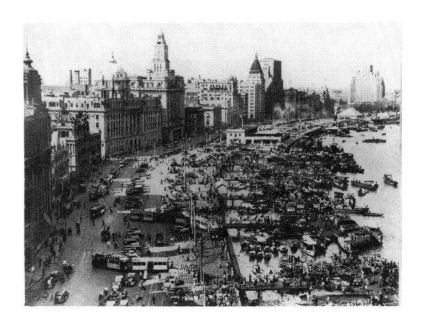

Manila Harbour 1940s

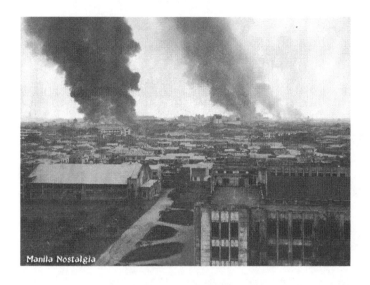

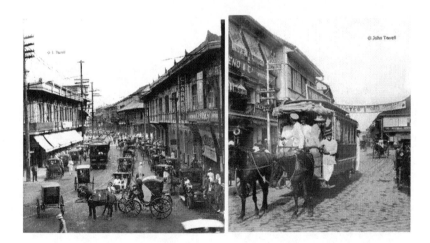

Manila city streets and bombings 1941

United States Army Sternberg Hospital Manila, Philippine

Upon reaching the city, we volunteered our services to the colonel in charge of the United States Army Sternberg Hospital. He happily accepted us duly registered and we spent our first night in the army hospital. At the time we signed in, wounded from Cavite Navy Yard were being brought to the hospital. Twelve Navy nurses, capable and efficient, accompanied the wounded. The chief nurse and I quickly became friends and I had the privilege of knowing her quite well.

From that time, until Japanese occupation three weeks later, we had breakfast at 6:30 a.m. and supper at 6:00 p.m. We ate in complete blackouts. Even flashlight bulbs had to be covered with black paper so that the hospital stayed in total blackout. The first night in the hospital we experienced great difficulty. The doctors and nurses groped their way through the corridor and along long tables. We could see nothing of our next-door neighbors and fellow workers. We needed all our attention, as it was required for us just to find a seat and a way to put food in our mouths. Even in this distress, we felt grateful for our army rations, even if we were not able to see what we were eating.

On December 22, the Japanese took over the Lingayen Gulf, and the United States and Filipino forces had to retreat into the Peninsula of Bataan and Corregidor, leaving the Allied civilians at the mercy of the Japanese. Manila and its vicinity were under Japanese air raids for three weeks before the outbreak of war and the Japanese occupation of the city. The Japanese captured five United States army posts: the United States Navy Yard; Santo Domingo Cathedral, the oldest and most revered in Manila; and also some parts of the walled city, which were all destroyed before capture.

261

I realized the situation was getting bad, and I wasn't sure I would be able to get on the ship that had been promised. I sent a telegram to my brother Neil McMillan on December 22, 1941: "Will call A1 Boston Mass No. transportation from Manila working in army hospital—Christmas greetings and love to all—return indefinite."

Manila was declared an open city, but that made no difference to the Japanese. The destruction of men in property still continued on just the same. On Christmas Eve, the hospital air raid siren blasted forth. Orders came to us following the hospital air raid siren that all ambulatory patients and staff should precede to the recently dug trenches on the hospital grounds. From 9:30 p.m. until around 2:30 a.m. we were obliged to spend Christmas Eve and Christmas morning in trenches wearing a helmet and gas mask, keeping still in place as the sirens screeched and the bombs exploded—*boom, boom*—all around us. It seemed an earth-shattering time for all of us and I must confess, in a few moments of terror, I was not sure if I would live to tell our story. But most of the time, we endured and kept our hope and faith that the Americans would arrive soon to save us.

On Christmas Day, the bombing continued. The nursing staff certainly persevered in doing justice to Uncle Sam's Christmas dinner despite the bombings. After each boom, the building trembled in shock in its foundation. The nurses jumped up from the table, threw themselves onto the floor or would flatten themselves against the wallboards, and every available spot been appropriated. My friend, Brunetta Kuelthau Gillet, was a dear and often told me her gratitude and how she appreciated my sense of humor under these difficult circumstances, as well as what an inspiration I was to all who met me. I just felt I was doing my job and was not there to win a popularity contest.

262

We all felt the same feelings, intense fear and desperation, as we huddled together in the trenches. We were all in the same immediate danger to oneself and one's friends close by and with each and every air raid brought us closer together.

Word came from Douglas MacArthur that American and Filipino officials would be evacuating to Corregidor. We knew that not only would our lives possibly be sacrificed at any moment, but also far worse: the death to innocent men, women, and children was happening everywhere in the country. Victims we had seen who might be obliged to spend years or possibly a lifetime disfigured or crippled. This site had become part of our reality when we saw plenty of the victims after each air raid. This tragic picture became a part of our daily experience and our heart wrenching reaction. The bombing continued and rocked the city and we became more disheartened.

The day following Christmas the bombing seemed almost continuous. During the last week of December 1941, the Standard Oil Company had been instructed by the United States government to destroy all their oil and gasoline supply. Some six million gallons burned up in smoke and flame during that week. The sky was ablaze with the fires every night, thick black smoke accompanied by towers of flames.

The greatest casualties of the civilian bombing took place during this time. Following each attack, the wounded were driven into the emergency department in the Army Hospital. The civilian casualties became so heavy, those in critical condition could get emergency dressings and be cared for, but all the other casualties were sent by car or truck to the Philippine General Hospital.

The room we were assigned to administer physiotherapy at Sternberg Hospital was adjacent to the operating room, which had been converted to a civilian emergency. The army physical therapist duties greatly increased along with the regular duties and I was also placed in charge of the surgical

263

supply room. Naturally, at such a time, the demand was very great, therefore all operating room nurses worked at replenishing surgical supplies and dressings every moment when not working in the operating room.

There was no time to feel or think, just to react to each new crisis that flew in front of us. It required quite a corps of workers to cope with the demand. The work was most efficiently handled. These abundant supplies over the course of the next few weeks were divided among the different departing units. Some nurses were asked to pack to go on the mercy ship carrying the critically wounded only, which left for Australia some were sent with the Bataan unit, and another group went to Corregidor.

It took three hours for the ambulances to transfer our wounded passengers to the ship leaving for Australia. Meanwhile, the people in the city scurried, looting took place and the gasoline dumps in Pandacan oil district were set on fire. I later found out that on their journey, the S.S. Mactan was fraught with great danger. The ship had to crisscross through a maze of mines just to leave Manila Bay and had to guide by a navy ship the whole way. The ship was also infested with insects and fraught by violent storms that tossed and drenched the patients on their cots. A fire broke out in the engine room and, for a time, those aboard prepared to abandon ship. By the grace of God, the ship arrived in the Sydney Harbor on January 27, 1942 with much fanfare. The wounded were taken immediately onto land and to the hospital.

On December 22, the Japanese arrived at Lingayen Gulf. Manila and MacArthur's troops held off the Japanese long enough so their units could retire into Bataan. The Americans and Filipinos flocked there for safety and the Japanese offered little resistance because McArthur declared Manila an open city to help save it from more destruction. This did not stop them from bombing Manila, though, until January 2, 1942.

264

Then on December 23, Japan took Wake Island, an American territory. Two days later, Hong Kong, a British colony, also fell to the Japanese. On December 29, Valdes returned to Manila on a secret mission to evacuate United States Army Forces in the Far East (USAFFE) troops from the Sternberg Hospital. Two hectic days followed. The Japanese had steadily bombed Manila and few ships were available. Other ships were sunk by mines, such as the S.S. Corregidor, which sank on December 16 and 17, and struck mines near Corregidor. Over 1,000 people drowned.

During the last wearisome week of 1941, the civilian casualties grew, and it became necessary for the remaining army and volunteer nurses to work well into the night, for there was so much extra work involved in the packing up the operating room and surgical equipment, surgical supplies, and dressing. The departing units carrying the wounded, each having it's own equipment, supplies, and the staff of doctors and nurses, covered for only a few more days.

They told us that we must evacuate the hospital because the Japanese were about to invade Manila and drop bombs on us. I telephoned the American Red Cross representative in Manila in the early evening of January, telling him of the valuable drug supplies and that more could be picked up at the army hospital, urging him to try to rescue at least some of those supplies rather than have them fall into the Japanese's hands. They replied that it was too late that evening to do anything. That response was more than we could take.

We decided to take the situation into our own hands. We convinced the owner of the Bay View Hotel to help us. He loaned us the largest hotel truck and his son came along to drive the truck. Three of us women loaded drugs and medical supplies from the army hospital by a flashlight, not knowing at that moment the enemy might come and find us.

265

In an hour or more the truck loaded the trucks well over half full, while the pockets of my khaki uniform bulged with a clinical thermometer and other small hospital necessities and around my neck were as many stethoscopes as I could carry. I felt as though we were starring in a spy picture show as we serendipitously entered the back gate of the hotel at midnight and immediately turned over all of the medical supplies to the local chapter of the Red Cross located in the Bay View Hotel

This global war destroyed happy dreams and became one of my greatest life challenges. By a twist of fate, I was now a victim of that war. I had taken a six-month leave prior to Pearl Harbor and was so close to never returning to China but returned despite being aware of all warning signals not to. Through it all, I still felt like I was one of the lucky ones. I had packed up many of my personal belongings, including all of my Chinese treasures, which I took with me on my last trip home. And so many people lost their homes, all their belongings, and even their lives.

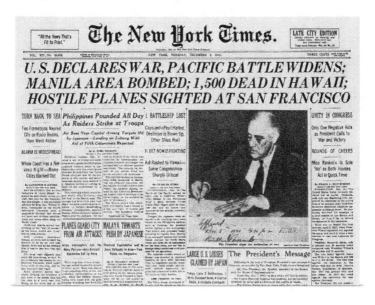

The New York Times December 9, 1941~ U.S. declares War

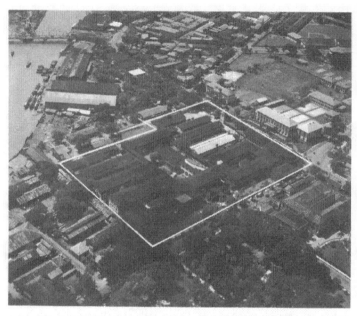

FIGURE 7.—Sternberg General Hospital, Manila, Philippine Islands, 1940.

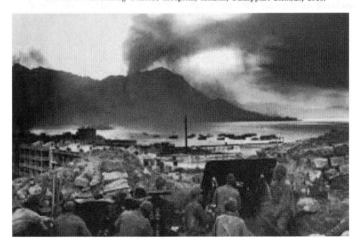

A Japanese artillery position at Braemar Hill, above North Point, in 1941

Not a Happy New Year

On December 31, all patients, doctors, and hospital staff were evacuated from the Sternberg Hospital. That evening the Mercy Ship, S.S. Mactan, loaded up as the sun was setting in the west. Only a few places in the world are blessed with such resplendent colors as the light of a Manila sunset. It was one of God and nature's most extravagant displays and provided a cinematic backdrop for the critically wounded being carried on their stretchers to the ship.   By sunrise the following morning, the ship slipped quietly away towards the south, to the shores of which they would sail to Sydney, Australia. Two hundred wounded soldiers, over half Americans, about 60 crewmembers, and medical personnel were on board.

The army hospital seemed like a graveyard after the sick, wounded, and the army medical nursing staff parted. A small civilian group remained, being transient, finding no place in the city to lay their heads. All hotels were crowded to overflowing with residents who were bombed out of their houses.

Other American and British residents left their homes fearing Japanese capture and moved to the hotels with a minimum of their personal effects. They preferred to share their fate along with the others facing the same situation. At the Sternberg Hospital, they placed all the names of the professional and civilian volunteers on the army payroll. For most of us, all our worldly possessions at the time comprised a suitcase filled with clothing and a regulation pay envelope that covered the period of service until New Year's Eve.

The Adjutant Army Official spoke on behalf of his chief who had left the previous day on S.S. Mactan and delivered heartfelt words of farewell. His voice registered emotion as he realized the seriousness of the situation. The small group of us who listened were deeply moved, as we were faced first hand with the eminent Japanese occupation.

268

The Japanese were only a few miles from the city. The news we heard from the local radio station was that the territory that had been under American jurisdiction for the last 40 years was now in the power of the Japanese.

In 1937, we had been in Peiping during the time of Japanese occupation following the so-called incident of Lu Kou Chou, which was a battle between the Republic of China's National Revolutionary Army and the Imperial Japanese Army. It was widely considered to have been the start of the Second Sino-Japanese War from 1937 to 1945. The Chinese still felt much sorrow and humiliation from that period and it was difficult for us to anticipate the challenges that would occur in this old revered city.

At the present instance, humiliation poured over the Manila citizens when they saw trains filled with Filipino, American soldiers, and civilians stranded, praying and waiting to be rescued, but no one had come. On January 2, 1942, the Japanese entered Manila and the remaining eleven army hospital nurses surrendered and were taken to Saint Scholastica Girls School with patients and other medical personnel.

Corregidor Still Stands

It seemed incredible to the people in Manila that the Japanese could capture their whole country in three weeks time. Tens of thousands of American dollars had been spent on public health, public schools, highways, and streets. Now all that had been built was under threat of the Japanese.

Commerce with the United States created and fostered sugar, copper, and other commodities. Much wealth had been created in mining of gold and other precious metals in the mountain regions north of Manila. Therefore, the radio announced every couple of hours, "Corregidor still stands!" in order to offer hope to the Filipino people.

269

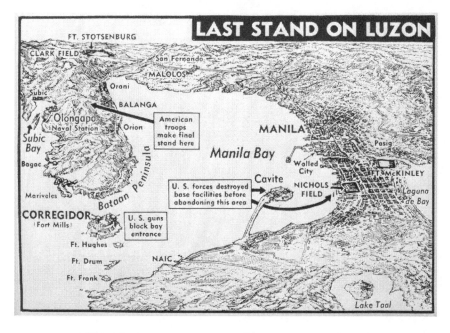

A United States Army Signal Corps map depicting the disposition of
U.S. forces in Luzon, Philippines, in 1942 (above) The Battle of Corregidor (below)

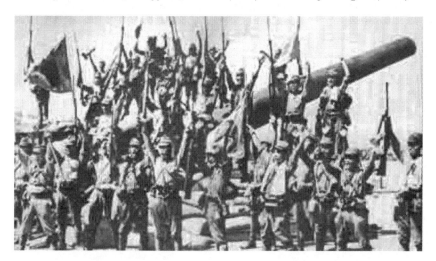

United States Army Troops Captured

I stood on the street with a sinking feeling in my stomach as I witnessed the faces of our American officers being driven in the captured American army trucks through the city of Manila on their way to the war prison camps. They looked tired, emaciated, and bedraggled. Our brave soldiers limped and shuffled down the main boulevard. For all the misery and suffering they endured, tears and smiles from the Filipinos lined the streets and were reciprocated by these men, even in defiance of armed Japanese guards. These officers' faces became pale, clothes tattered rags, but one could tell their spirits were neither crushed nor broken.

The soldiers tried their best to respond to the enthusiastic readings of the friendly Filipinos lining Dewey Boulevard, despite the Japanese guards with fixed bayonets on them. The Filipinos threw packages of cigarettes and cheered as the soldiers trudged along on their foot sores, exhausted from the inhumane treatment they received from exposure and lack of nourishment. These poor fellows were too sick to even respond except for faint smile recognition or gratitude for the wholehearted sincerest cries of the crowds.

Many civilian Filipinos on the streets attempting to help the soldiers were struck across the face or had their arms, body, or legs prodded with rifle bats. The Japanese guards moved along marching soldiers with bayonets pointed for action at the slightest sign of intimacy between the soldiers and the people on the street.

I had grown tired and weary, became very ill, and was granted a temporary sick leave for a few days. I was sent to the home of a training nurse near the city. She was one of the finest women and it has been my good fortune to know her. She had been acting as chief nurse at the Steinberg Hospital before the Japanese occupation. She went about her duties with a smile and always had a word of cheer for patients and nurses alike. She was indeed a benediction in her distribution of friendly charity and encouragement.

271

Her kindness, understanding heart, and skill endeared her to all. During the first weeks of occupation under the constant strain of night and day bombings, at the worst moments, what a blessing she was to thousands of wounded soldiers laying in the hospital beds built into the stonewalls of the army hospital beneath Corregidor rock. The entire rock reverberated day and night. It was like constant thunder clapping around them, each bomb clapping, then wrecking and tearing at the nerves of patients and staff. Above it all was this unknown heroine as she filled her daily tasks with helmet and gas mask at alert, fearless and courageous at all times.

While I convalesced, we learned that Japanese officers entered the lobby of the Bay View Hotel in Manila, located on the corner of Dewey Street and UN Avenue. The street had been a showcase for the city and was a bustling area designed in Spanish Colonial motif with wide-open spaces where acacias lined the sidewalks. The High Commissioner's office, the Plaza Militar, the Polo Club, Night Club, casinos, and an expensive corporate residence were all here. The hotel's owner, Dr. Kneedler, bought the hotel in 1934 and it became known for its cocktail hours.

Sadly, the owners were obliged to place a signature on a paper, which turned over the hotels and its equipment to the Japanese. That hotel and others, in addition to apartment houses, were obliged to do the same thing. All of the American civilians from Bataan had been captured by truck and taken to the Santo Tomas Internment Camp, which had extreme overcrowding and near starvation. The prisoners experienced great trials. They suffered for weeks from a shortage of water and food. The only food they had for subsistence was a few canned goods left in their outfits. All registered a high fever and were suffering from dysentery, malaria, and marked nutritional deficiency. Practically all of the internees suffered from malnutrition.

Then all the American, British, and Dutch citizens who had been living in Manila and the surrounding country were rounded up in the first week of 1942 and brought to internment camps. I was among those who were captured and left to wait among many who were stranded.

272

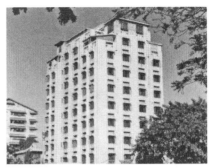

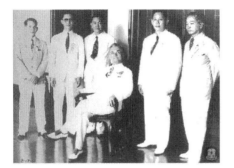

THE DAILY TIMES-NEWS

MANILA IS LOST

**Capital Says
Loss Serious,
U.S. Fights On**

**Naval Base At Cavite
Falls To Japan Today;
Battle Is Continuing**

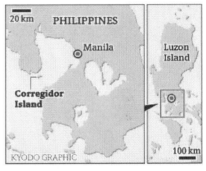

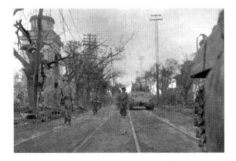

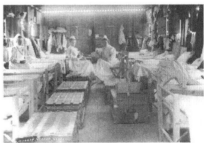

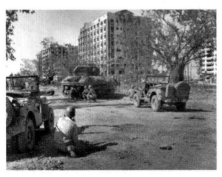

The Tribune

BATAAN COMPLETELY OCCUPIED BY JAPANESE

Japanese Forces Take Cebu

15 Generals Among War Prisoners

Japanese Flag Planted In Cebu City

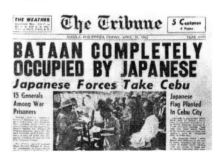

Manila seized by Japanese, Bay View Hotel, Quezon cabinet, map, destruction, and Sternberg Hospital

Most people had little warning regarding this notice; some had no warning at all. There was a great deal of looting in the local shops and vacated homes at this time, and we were totally shocked and confused as to what fate awaited us.

United States High Commissioner Francare by Sears' house on the waterfront was the scene of much Japanese activity during the first night of Japanese occupancy. Officers on motorcycles charged into the drive in front of the house from midnight until the early morning hours and the entire house was flooded with light.

Along Main Street in the city, Japanese commandeered all parked cars, they even entered public and private garages, and did the same thing: a small white flag with a red sun was left on every windshield to signify Japanese position. Dewey Boulevard was ablaze with light all night as the Japanese took over the city.

During this time, many people were interrogated, including high-ranking members of the Shanghai Municipal Police (SMP), journalists, radio announcers, newspaper editors, bankers, importers, society organizers, merchants, hotel employees, and engineers, among others. Torture was standard and prisoners were held without recourse for days or months. Those who survived and were released generally emerged with serious injuries, infections, and mental or emotional trauma.

On January 4, 1942, the Japanese's greatest enemies—British, American, and Dutch nationalities—were ordered to register with the Japanese authorities, and their assets frozen or confiscated. They were made to wear red armbands marked with a letter to signify their nationality. The British wore armbands marked with "B" and the Americans wore the letter "A." All civilians were given orders to register with the Swiss Consulate to obtain identity cards, and curfews were instituted.

Mobile checkpoints organized by the Japanese Pao Chia were erected around the city to search for anti-Japanese agitators. Residents caught up in these searches could be detained for hours or days without food or water, leading many to carry provisions with them every time they left the house. If arrested, they could be sent to Bridge House, a notorious interrogation and detention center set up by the Japanese.

274

A MESSAGE
TO THE FILIPINO PEOPLE

The determination of the Filipino people to continue fighting side by side with the United States until victory is won has in no way been weakened by the temporary reverses suffered by our arms. We are convinced that our sacrifices will be crowned with victory in the end and in that conviction we shall continue to resist the enemy with all our might.

Japanese military forces are occupying sections of the Philippines comprising only one third of our territory. In the remaining areas constitutional government is still in operation under my authority.

I have no direct information concerning the veracity of the news broadcast from Tokyo that a Commission composed of some well-known Filipinos has been recently organized in Manila to take charge of certain functions of civil government. The organization of such a commission, if true, can have no political significance not only because it is charged merely with purely administrative functions but also because the acquiescence by its members to serve in the Commission was evidently for the purpose of safeguarding the welfare of the civilian population and can, in no way, reflect the sentiments of the Filipino towards the enemy. Such sentiments are still those I have repeatedly expressed in the past: Loyalty to America and resolute resistance against the invasion of our territory and liberties.

MANUEL L. QUEZON,
President of the Philippines.

United States Army Forces in the Far East
HEADQUARTERS FIRST REGULAR DIVISION
In the Field

January 20, 1942

Dear President Quezon,

I want to thank you for your personal letter which has been read to all the troops under my command.

Since December 29, 1941, my Division has been manning the battle position. On that date every man was **exhorted to hold his** ground. On the 16th of January, 1942, these troops with that gallant Troop "G" from the valiant 26th Cavalry, attacked the enemy in Moron and drove him north of the Batalan River with heavy casualties on his part, resulting in captured materiel and identification of the enemy units. General Wainright tells me that this is the first instance where Filipino troops attacked first. Heretofore, Filipinos have only counterattacked.

It should hearten you to know that all men of this Division, Americans and Filipinos alike, are fighting the foe at this very moment for all that their lives are worth ignoring all handicaps in training, equipment and lack of air support.

Respectfully yours,

FIDEL V. SEGUNDO
Brigadier General
Commanding

President Manuel L. Quezon

To be read

HEADQUARTERS, FIRST INFANTRY, P.C.

In the Field, Km. Post 189.8
18 January 1942

His Excellency,
Hon. Manuel L. Quezon
President of the Commonwealth of the Philippines
Bataan.

My dear Mr. President:

I wish to acknowledge with extreme gratification the receipt yesterday of your inspiring message of the 15th and to convey to Your Excellency the warm and enthusiastic reception accorded to it by each and every member of my command.

Again, we pledge our unswerving loyalty and firm determination, with the constant prayer that, exerting to the utmost our combined abilities, we will not be found lacking. The 1st Infantry Regiment, PC, is right behind Your Excellency and the High Command as one man, so rest assured, sir, that in this, our fight for a most righteous cause, we will do our share faithfully and will be ready to die in the attempt if need be.

To us, there is no hardship too great that we cannot endure; no obstacle too strong that we cannot surmount. As true Filipino soldiers, we shall remain fast to our sworn duty and continue to hold, and hold, and hold some more, as is wont us and as long as we are called upon to do so.

We are all fully confident, sir, that, God willing, with America's promised aid, our beloved Philippines will survive this difficult ordeal, this baptism of hell forced upon all of us, and together, under your leadership, emerge victorious as a nation, reborn - truly great and deserving of a peaceful and prosperous existence under Far Eastern skies.

Please accept our warmest regards and best wishes for your continued good health.

We remain, sir, always at your service.

Devotedly yours,

N. N. CASTAÑEDA
Colonel, 1st Infantry, PC
Regimental Commander.

THE WEATHER

Yesterday's Max.: 94.0 C., or
94.1 F., at 3:35 P. M. Min.:
93.1 C. or 79 F., at 6:45 A. M.

The Tribune

5 Centavos
4 Pages

YEAR XVIII   MANILA, PHILIPPINES, FRIDAY, MAY 8, 1942   NUMBER 38

CORREGIDOR FALLS

General Wainwright Orders Entire USAFFE to Surrender

Troops Must Disarm, Give Up in 4 Days

Instructions
To Officers, Men
Read Over Radio

By Eutorio del Rosario and
A. J. Malay of the Tribune staff

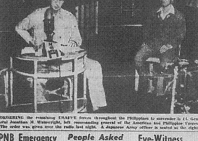

ORDERING the remaining USAFFE forces throughout the Philippines to surrender is Lt. General Jonathan M. Wainwright, left commanding general of the American and Philippine forces. The order was given over the radio last night. A Japanese Army officer is seated at the right.

Japan Forces Occupy Entire Stronghold

Tokyo Imperial
Headquarters Makes
Announcement

TOKYO, May 7 (Domei)—Imperial Headquarters announced at 3:30 o'clock this afternoon that Japanese army and navy forces succeeded in landing on Corregidor Island in the face of enemy fire at 11:15 o'clock last Tuesday night, May 5, and by 6 o'clock in the morning of Thursday, May 7, had completely occupied Corregidor and other islands at the other islands in Manila Bay.

PNB Emergency Notes Banned

People Asked To Display Nippon Flag

Eye-Witness Tells of "Fall"

Wainwright Surrenders

(Continued on page 3)

Army Spokesman Says Fall Of Corregidor Significant

Mayor Guinto Urges People To Welcome Commander-in-Chief

San Francisco Has Raid Alert

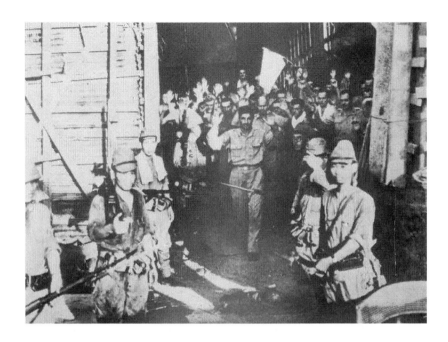

U.S. troops surrendering to Japanese soldiers at Corregidor Island, Philippines, May 1942

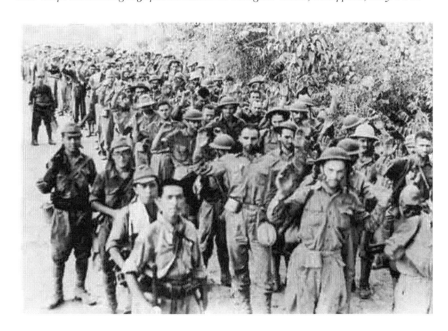

COPY

*Pysiotherapy
McMillan*

orig us war Dept

August 3, 1942

Miss Agnes M. Pearce
China Medical Board, Inc.,
49 West 49th Street,
New York City, New York

Dear Miss Pearce:

    The Provost Marshal General has directed me to inform you
that this office has received official information that the following
are interned by Japan and that they are "well": Miss Ethel Robinson,
Doctor Frank E. Whitacre, and Miss Margaret Wyne. The place of internment is not known.

    This office has also received official information that Miss
Mary McMillan has been interned by Japan. Miss McMillan sends the
message "well---regards to all."

    You may communicate with them by following the instructions
on the inclosed directions for sending ordinary mail.

    When their names appear on further information received by
this office, you will be notified.

             Sincerely yours,

             Howard F. Bresee,
             Lt. Col., C. M. P.,
             Chief, Information Bureau.

2 incls.
  info. cirs.

14

THERE WAS STILL HOPE

Santo Tomas Internment Camp

O n January 5, 1942, my friend from the Sternberg Hospital, Josephine Bell, and I spent our first night in the Santo Tomas Internment Camp. Our new home was housed at the Manila University, which was located on a 65-acre compound. We had been told that we should all pack clothing and food for three days and Japanese soldiers would pick us up. Like cattle, they drove us in army trucks from the hotel in states of bewilderment and confusion.

We discovered close to 4,000 people starkly deposited behind university barred gates with the fence topped with shards of broken glass to prevent escape. Hundreds of Japanese soldiers guarded the prisoners, which was an entirely shocking experience to all. In fact, the whole occurrence seemed like a nightmare.

Chaos awaited us on our arrival. They split the women and men up and shoved us into classrooms in groups of 30 and 40. We each wrestled with a mixture of emotions of fear, nervousness, anxiety, and terror. There was a part of us that believed this situation was temporary and the Americans would save us soon, and another part of us had little hope we would be saved.

However, very soon the nightmare we thought was unreal, turned to a harsh reality. My first week of internment, a cold hard cement floor was to be my only sleeping place. Then, with good fortune, a group of three other women invited me join them under one mosquito netting on an inverted wood filing cabinet, which became the only bed I knew for many months.

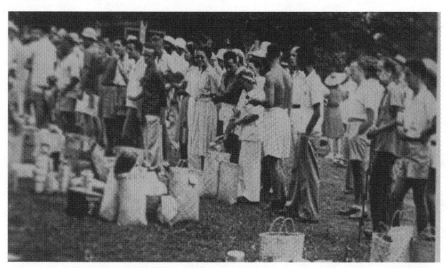

Internees at the Santo Tomas camp in Manila arrived with just the belongings they could carry from their outside residences. (Courtesy: Jim Crosby)

There was a lack of food, of bed or bedding, clothing, and most importantly, one's freedom. Everyone had to live off their own food, which they had packed. Some servants were allowed to visit twice a day to bring prisoners food, clothes, laundry, bedding, and other supplies. After the first week, the internees were given two meals a day, wheat or corn, bread, and coffee at 7:00 a.m. and dinner at 4:30 p.m.

In the first month, there were almost 4,000 internees, mostly American and British, with some Australians and Norwegians, of which 700 were children thrown in to live together. At first, the Japanese commandant allowed local Filipinos to bring supplies to the internees but little by little they were told to stop.

284

The one blessing under the horrifying circumstances was that Japanese allowed us to create our own self-government. Within a very short time an executive committee was elected. They created other committees to help with various needs as they became apparent. The committees were housed under an executive board, and consisted of purchasing, bathroom, educational, religious, secretarial, camp news, entertainment, building, social welfare, sanitary squad, police force, and kitchen squad. These groups all worked through the executive board and the chairman acted as a liaison officer between the internees and the Japanese commandment. This male internee was responsible to the Japanese military authorities that had their quarters in the city. They had the last word on the final decision.

The executive board supplied each room monitor with the request slip. Upon application, a slip could be obtained, filled out by the internee, and handed over for approval from the executive board before the application was made to the Japanese Commandments for a signature. An incoming package had to correspond to the request and be checked first by the distributing group and then censored by the Japanese before being delivered into the hands of the internees.

The executive board headed all of the operations of the camp. They made it a custom that before authorizing the purchasing committee to buy supplies, they had to obtain the necessary funds or be assured that these funds would be forthcoming. As a temporary measure, the Filipino Red Cross had to advance funds, in addition to many beds, mattresses, and considerable bedding for the hospital. Also, many mattresses and mosquito netting was purchased for those internees who had no way of purchasing them.

At a certain point, the Japanese stopped the cash allowance that was being given from the Filipino Red Cross to their American Allies because we were considered the enemies of the Japanese. The average Filipino loved the Americans and were loyal and interested in helping in every possible way. The loyalty and devotion of many of the Filipinos showed a great tribute to American sovereignty in the Philippines. The International Red Cross assumed financial aid for some time, but the Japanese also stopped that.

Later when the Japanese got around to printing paper money in Manila without gold behind it, creating money was without cost to them. We were given 35 cents per person a day to keep us fed. This included kitchen equipment, garbage pails, wheel barrels, toilet paper, medicine for the hospital, and every item used in the camp. Therefore, 35 cents per person might be reduced to about twenty cents a day, per person, for food.

Internees who had homes were allowed to have their household effects, clothing, and food sent to the camp. Transient prisoners were unable to indulge in such privileges. A shed was erected by the camp carpenter near the front gate and sectioned off as a mail office letter and customs.

The American representative checked on each package before Japanese censorship, then one intern delivered the package or letters to the internees. The camp elected a purchasing committee and purchased all camp food and supplies. These interns were allowed to go to the city daily for this express purpose only.

All camp rules and regulations instigated by the executive board had to be submitted to the Japanese commandment for approval. He was established in a commodious office in the main building and had a large secretarial staff comprised of Japanese and qualified internees.

There were also Japanese guards under a separate sheet. These guards paraded around the grounds every day and every night. In the early days of internment, a guard came into the dormitory after people went to bed. They would use a flashlight and flash it into the faces of prisoners lying in bed, on mattresses, or on the floor.

286

Should the number counted not agree with the Japanese count in the room, then everyone was commanded to get up. They counted everyone in the room again or lined them up out in the corridor according to the particular fancy of a guard on duty.

Later, they changed this procedure. Each room was assigned its own individual monitor. The monitor had to count each person listed. They called roll early in the morning and again at sunset and were responsible to the Japanese that no one was missing. Two Japanese guards paraded the corridors all night.

American volunteer police decided it would give the women a feeling of security if American patrols also kept a night ritual. So, night shifts were arranged, which indeed was a very kind gesture on the part of the internee volunteer police. The women appreciated this nightly visual, which gave us a much greater sense of security.

We tried our best to normalize our daily lives by creating our own small city by order, a structure, and a sense of community, as a way to survive the chaos and uncertainty we had been forced into. Four weeks before the opening of the camp kitchen, our small group was obliged to wash off some stone steps on one of the buildings each time before eating. Water for washing or drinking had to be carried some distance from a pump and, of course, the usual queue each time. Then wood had to be picked up from the grounds and a fire built before the primitive cooking could be undertaken. Old tin cans picked up from the garbage being washed then scoured with earth, to be used as cooking utensils.

Fortunately, my friends and I considered ourselves lucky to have anything to cook at all because we were not from the city, and transients had no such an opportunity to receive any help from the outside. We would have starved if it had not been for the good heartedness of a British man who kindly interested himself in our welfare. He kindly shared the food his Filipina secretary brought to him twice a week.

287

The education committee gathered together a group of professional teachers and organized regular classes from nursery school to college matriculation. These classes met at odd places, chiefly in the grounds but also on the steps of buildings, which were not used as regular thoroughfares. The required matriculation standards were maintained throughout all grades.

At the end of the first month, the committee's interned schoolteachers set up classes again in the university's chemistry labs. They taught every subject except for American history, which was forbidden by the Japanese. The kids didn't much enjoy going to school, but it passed the time. At times, some kids despaired that the internment would never end. For distraction, they played cops and robbers for hours.

Workers in every field seemed imbued with the spirit to overcome all obstacles. They were determined to make the best of what they had to work with. The educational committee was allowed to bring from the outside certain necessary textbooks and frugal school supplies to meet some of their educational needs. Books from ten school libraries were brought into camp. It was a very helpful thing for the children to be able to carry on their schooling even amid overwhelming difficulties. It was a blessing for teachers to have an incentive to accomplish such a difficult task. Proficient instructors for the adult courses often commended the education committee for planning lecture courses. Almost every subject from language to science was included in the program of courses.

One month's time elapsed between internment and the opening of the camp kitchen. The main body of the kitchen squad did not go into action for a month following the opening of Santo Tomas. A smaller group was sufficient to prepare food for the children in the early days before the main kitchen was built. From day one, the children received cracked wheat and coco. The Filipino Red

Cross served coffee to the adults from 7:00 a.m. to 9:00 a.m. every morning and donated food.

The camp kitchen was not able to function until the equipment was purchased and installed. The kitchen squad was composed of cooks, dishwashers, serving attendance, and garbage collectors, all of whom waited to take on their respective duties when the kitchen opened. The internees' skilled carpenters and plumbers did the labor of kitchen construction, equipment, and installation. They served food cafeteria-style from large food containers when the kitchen was ready to function. The serving team ladled out hot food twice daily, accompanied by smiles, and very often, a word of good cheer.

Long cues waited every morning and every evening. Sometimes instead of coffee, they served hot tea at breakfast. The morning cereal was a gift of the American Red Cross and the most satisfactory food of the day. In the early days, a small supply of milk and sugar was also served. Powdered milk supply was limited and considered necessary and saved for the babies and the children in camp.

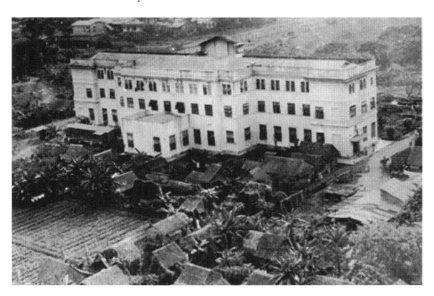

Ariel view of San Tomas Internment Camp under Japanese occupation

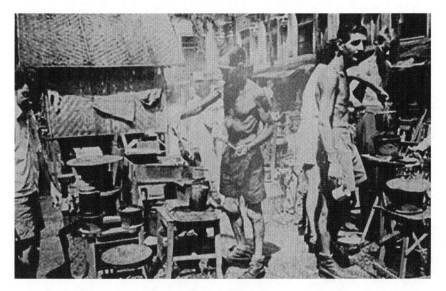

Shanties in the camps with makeshift cooking platforms

About the time of the opening of the camp kitchen, the purchasing committee procured a very large Ringling Circus tent. This proved to be very excellent protection from the blazing Oriental sun. Benches from the classrooms were placed under the tent top, which provided a nice dining room for the two daily meals. Also, various groups of school children assembled there between meals for classes.

On the second floor of the main building, 470 women showered in one bathroom, which had only five toilets, one of which was always out of order, three showers, and two washbowls. It was a sad-looking bathing and toilet facility.

The women internees each took daily schedules for bathroom duty. The bathroom monitor stood by the door at her appointed hour and handed each person four pieces of toilet paper. Later, this amount had to be decreased due to the shortage of paper. Her duty also included a check-up on line crashing and was sure the toilets

290

were properly flushed. Flushing was not a simple matter. For the toilets to flush, a chain was pulled as a hit or miss.

When the purchasing committee was allowed to procure materials, plumbers and builders speedily added showers and toilets in the camp hospital and main building, which had formerly been used as college executive offices. The building committee was able to supplement the previous one shower with two additional showers. Even so, with three showers and five toilets, one was always out of order and two washable basins were not adequate for 470 women and children.

Three couples were required to occupy all three showers at the same time, so there was no possibility of privacy, even in the showers, which had no curtains between the showers. They closed the bathroom each day for one hour for cleaning purposes. Disinfectant was used freely by the male cleaning squad daily.

The men shared a funny story, told of a young bank clerk who said he got the greatest satisfaction at having his bank boss hand

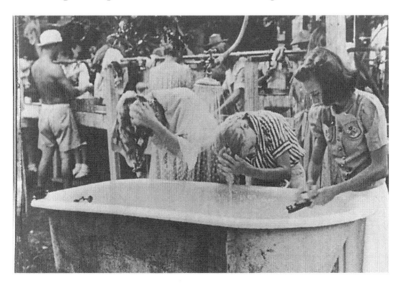

Internees washing their hair and clothes

him over the allotted toilet paper and even a greater kick when they worked on the toilet squad together.

Everyone was equal at the camp. We all began at square one and it did not matter if you were rich, educated, famous, or beautiful. We were all prisoners of war and the Japanese did not care and treated us worse than animals. One president of the bank replied to his employee's remark, "Well sir, it seems strange to see you hand out toilet paper." To which the bank manager replied, "Oh that's nothing, I'm quite accustomed to handing out deposit slips."

Sanitary Squad

The sanitary squad did a really magnificent piece of work, guarding against epidemics and keeping flies and mosquitoes in control. Five hundred men had been assigned to this group and I thought not too many for the class of task, it needed to be done. Public health doctors and engineers headed this work assisted by professionals and businessman.

The dormitories and kitchen swarmed with flies and mosquitoes at the beginning of camp life. By means of cleverly devised flytraps near each cover garbage pail in the kitchen and on the grounds, we killed thousands of flies every day. Children were invited to join the fly contest. They distributed locally made fly swatters among the youngsters. Boys and girls joined in competitive groups and rewards were offered to the highest fly killers.

To prevent mosquito breeding in exposed water, they used oil spray, flint guns, and flip powder which was provided to each room monitor for daily use in all of the internees' living quarters. The sanitary squad also instigated rules to cope with the bedbug situation. The group cleaned each room and bare dry and wet mopped every mattress for those who were fortunate up to possess one. Each bed had to be carried out into the sunlight regularly and taken back inside at night. All mosquito nettings had to be kept thoroughly clean at all times. They sprayed Insecticides regularly on walls' woodwork, mattresses, and beds springs.

Troughs were built for washing clothes and extra drains added to accommodate thousands of individuals. The sanitary committee purchased covered garbage pails, which were placed in convenient positions. All garbage had to be sanitarily disposed of daily within the camp precincts. This called for men to collect, burn, and bury garbage twice daily. A necessary but quite a difficult task, for sanitary disposal of such large quantities of garbage required plenty of brain and muscle power. It was a lot of work to be a prisoner of war.

Morale improved from the weekly check-ups made by members of the sanitary squad to all dormitories and bathrooms. The sanitary group fostered rivalry for the cleanest and neatest room. Every room was listed and a gold star presented by the monitor for the best room each week. One gold star was given to the men's dormitory and one for the women's. The earned star was then posted proudly on the room door. This small gold star not only inspired pride in cleanliness, but it also helped make life more livable with so large and diverse a group of people showering in one dormitory.

Even so simple a grade school scheme as a gold star contest brought considerable enthusiasm and interest among the internees. There was one of the men's rooms that excelled above all others in gold stars. They worked together early and late to keep their room tops with the gold star rating. They were as proud as a lot of youngsters winning a schoolyard race. The beds or mattresses on the floor were so close that one could touch one's neighbor on either side. In one instance, seven unrelated women slept under one mosquito net. It would seem that seven cots as closely placed as possible for months on end was hardly a kind of sleeping condition, even from the sanitary standpoint, that any human being should have to endure.

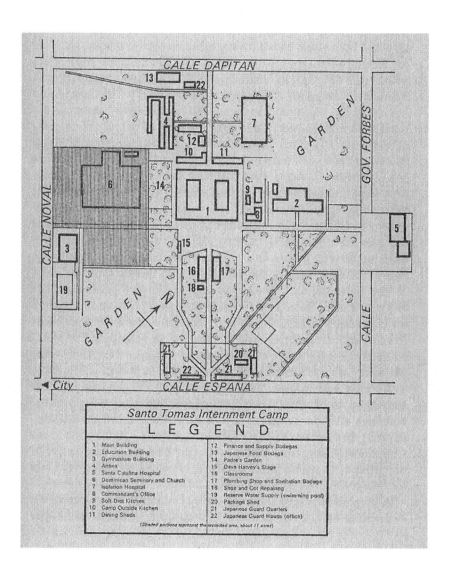

Santa Tomas Internment Camp Map

Adjusting to a New Life as Prisoner

The internment camp was an enormous physical and psychological adjustment that most people found difficult to take in the days order. The mental and emotional feelings of insecurity, both financial and physical, were not easy to accept. They were only made worse because families had been divided, the men in one building and the women and children in another.

With a heterogeneous group of several thousand people, all forced together had to live with inevitable personality adjustments and sucking up strong emotions that must be buried inside us because a Japanese guard could kill an internee at any moment if we looked at them the wrong way. The complete lack of privacy was a hardship, perhaps the hardest. It's a wonder things went on as well as they did.

In our past daily lives, we had taken for granted comfortable chairs and adequate lighting; in camp life, however, these luxuries did not exist. The shortage of bathing and toilet facilities was indeed a trial. In a tropical climate like Manila, it is imperative that cleanliness of the strictest order is followed. This resulted in long lines of women night and day in order to comply with the necessary demands. The average loss of weight reached around 25 pounds. In many instances, this loss of weight resulted in lower resistance and people soon became very ill.

Intestinal troubles, dysentery, and dengue fever were prevalent, and also malaria among the internees. In the rainy season, there was a great deal of arthritic issues due to the dampness, diet, and poor housing conditions. Standing in lines an hour for two meals twice a day became extremely tiring. The personal responsibility of daily living was no easy task.

Due to malnutrition and these ailments, internees united once again to supplement the starchy diet of rice and wheat. They planted gardens of weeds and wild plants to put in the broth stews. It only made a slight difference, but each small change brought us hope, and this helped us to keep moving forward in spite of the tragic circumstances.

Camp Operations

We created a secretarial and operations committee, which had quite a staff of stenographers, clerks, and assistants. The secretarial office became the busiest place of camp activities. All internees' appointments first presented to the executive board the orders for action. Several Americans who were conversant in Japanese, also acted as interpreters in important communications with our capturers.

For events such as the death of a relative; instances of eye trouble, which could not be cared for adequately in the camp or camp hospital; or critical conditions which required immediate operation, the head of the committee referred those people to the hospital director, a Japanese doctor, and then the executive committee for action before being presented to the commandment for his approval and signature.

Each internee listed in the comprehensive record file was kept up-to-date in the secretary's office. A weekly check-up by the hospital staff was made to see that each internee had been working in the field of labor, profession, business, household, or academic studies or the arts, for which they were specially trained. The files were the Japanese property and guarded by them day and night.

The camp internees assembled a new staff headed up by an associated press correspondent who had been selected by the executive board. Items of interest to the internees' camp of the regulations, as well as jokes, found their way into the weekly mimeograph sheets, which were given out for free. Later, one of the
camp artists cleverly colored some drawings in a three-month small mimeographed issue. The larger published pamphlets became very popular among the internees because of the clever jokes and cartoons. The larger issues were sold and could be purchased for 25 cents a copy.

Many of our greatest afflictions, like the rainy season, which lasted for many weeks, proved excellent material for cartoons. The British came in for their share in the fun poking. One memorable drawing was of an Englishman balancing on top of free floating barrel—wearing high boots and a hat perched at a rakish angle— calling out to a passer-by, who stood in the water up to his knees, saying, "I say old chap, a bit dampish, eh?" With the usual true sportsmanship of the British, they accepted it, apparently with impersonal relish.

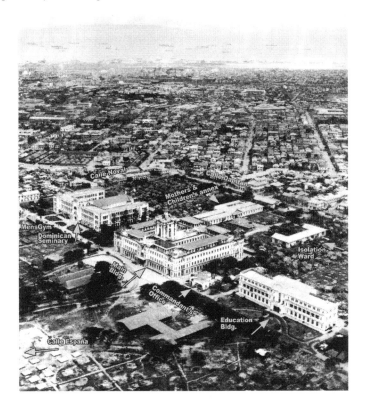

Santa Tomas Interment Buildings Map

Internee Hospital

The hospital committee established a camp hospital in one of the former science buildings of the university, selected as the best possible place. I was chosen as one of the leads on this committee. Within a week of our internment, the camp hospital designated the former college building of metallurgy and meteorology. Cabinets containing specimens of metal and of meteors therefore decorated the hospital walls.

The Filipino Red Cross provided the hospital with 80 beds and our camp hospital staff composed of qualified doctors and graduate nurses. A daily clinic connected with the hospital was open to internees who needed medical service attention. Due to sleeping on cement floors or classroom benches, many without even mattresses, it was physically hard upon those who formerly had suffered from back weakness.

Psychologically, many endured the shock of the suddenness of the Japanese invasion and the loss of tangible and intangible possessions, which also led to reasonable mental stress. So, some of those patients arrived at a makeshift hospital. Very shortly after the hospital opened, every bed was occupied, and our daily clinic kept on growing. Doctors were on call at every hour of the day. Volunteer nurses and orderlies worked tirelessly day and night. A long line of patients waited to be seen, and the nurses and staff became very busy with the complaints.

Patients were soon asked to come by appointment, much as in the city hospitals. The doctors only performed minor operations, as no operating room nor facility existed. The director of the hospital, after consultation with the Japanese doctor, was granted permission from the commandment for emergency operations and sent to the Philippine General Hospital, which was under Japanese control.

In the earlier days, many of the drugs used in the hospital and clinic had been looted from the United States Army Sternberg Hospital just previous to the Japanese occupation; and in other parts of the building, the staff often heard dormant cries from the 80 occupied beds, but the staff of doctors, nurses, and orderlies dutifully continued their work to help all of the internees who suffered with meds or not.

The hardship was increased, as only one bathroom with two toilets was all the hospital provided. A few months later, the committee added two more toilets and additional showers, which made the hospital hygiene at least physically a little more bearable for all concerned.

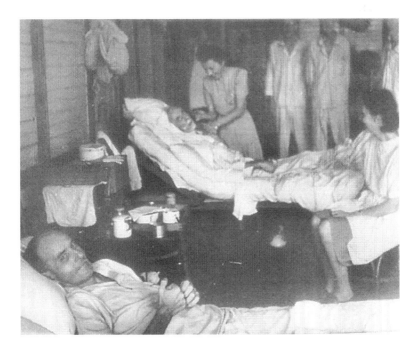

Army nurse Gwendolyn Henshaw works in the camp hospital ward

Army Nurses in Camp

Some nurses after the siege of Bataan reached the United States by plane. The rest of the army nurses arrived at the camp from the fall of Corregidor. These women were not allowed by the Japanese to have any communication with other internees for many weeks. Our enemy imprisoned them in houses at Santa Catalina, a building across the road and beyond the original camp limits.

Several months later, a new entrance opened from Santo Tomas Internment Camp to Santa Catalina. The original camp hospital was transferred to this larger building and 150 beds replaced the 80 beds. At the time, they placed the army nurses in charge of the hospital.

The commandment issued a letter to the internees requesting people who desired to go to Shanghai to sign on the dotted line. To most of the internees at Santo Tomas, this invitation was shrouded with distrust. They discredited any possible good intention from the Japanese. In any case, the overwhelming majority considered those who did sign as crazy or foolhardy, to say the least.

Some doctors, nurses, and orderlies who served in the camp hospital signed on to take the trip. It seemed as if repatriation from Shanghai was more likely than from the Manila territory, which had flown the stars and stripes for the past 40 years. The hospital needed to enlarge its bed capacity, and its clinical services required larger quarters. This seemed a good time to make these changes.

They transferred directorship of the camp hospital to a well known American doctor who had previously been in practice in Manila for years. The responsibility of the nursing services was taken over by 60 nurses and the small group of navy nurses. The original group of hospital personnel deserved great credit for the organization and functioning of our little internment hospital until that time. Thousands of internees had received the best medical advice and as much of other hospital facilities as possible under the unbearable conditions at hand. Most of the doctors and nurses refused to lose their spirits because they believed that it would give the Japanese satisfaction to break the internees' morale.

300

They took pride in spite of the tragic circumstances and rallied to keep up the community spirit.

I set up my physiotherapy shop in a small room in the science building next to the space reserved for the daily clinic. I put my knowledge and clever hands to perform miracles on patients with hot water, basins, and bath towels with a few pills. As my work spread amongst the camp, our department became swamped. I asked Miss Martha Hill to help me. Robert Slaves, a bright high school boy trained in first aid, became my right-hand man. We had fun along with our work, and people would stick their heads in to see what we were laughing about. Helping with patients' backs and arthritis from sleeping on the cold cement, pulled muscles, painful feet, infected bed bug bites, and rashes, all manner of aches and pains, were brought to us every day. They would leave feeling better after half an hour with us.

The Police Squad

The police squad found that their problems grew as rules and regulations were instigated for this and that offense. They did not often report minor misdemeanors, such as walking too close to a roped off section or failing to bow sufficiently low to Japanese gardens near the gate. A stern reprimand from the volunteer internee police on duty usually sufficed because the internees were walking on eggshells and living in fear most of the time.

More serious misdemeanors or rule breaking brought about the tension in this so-called brig. The rule breaker was called before the chief of police and his staff for their discussion regarding time of detention. Men and women were warehoused in separate rooms but it was by no means unusual to hear about expectant mothers in the camp. The head of the hospital stated the cost for the suggested sick leave. I had to pass all "leave of absence" paperwork.

There were too many requests for a leave of absence for prospective mothers, so the prospective fathers were to be considered offenders. They decided that the fathers would be punished in a brig for the term of the mother's pregnancy.

301

Religious and Social Committee

The religious and social committee assumed the most difficult task in the community. Ordained priests worked with pastors and social leaders, all of whom worked harmoniously, for the religions and social interest of the internees. People were passionate about their religions and set in their ways, so finding common ground between the three main religions was no easy feat. One section of the grounds, located between the main buildings in the University Roman Catholic chapel, known as the "father's garden," was kept apart for religions services on Sundays.

This committee also planned lectures and open forms. A church choir of male and female vocals held the regular practices in this place. There was a day and time set for each sects of religious services and the internees peacefully complied.

Sports

The social directors committee planned sports and games for the younger people. Weekly community competition became very popular and included both the young and older people. Informal dances, for the teenagers only, were naturally fun and very much needed. The children on the whole suffered least because the adults provided them with three meals a day instead of the two given to the adults. Lessons in the open air, games and sports, lots of play, without the insecurity felt by their parents hovering over them, tended to make life in the internment camp not such a bad thing for the younger fry.

Entertainment

The entertainment committee was comprised of quite a number of professional entertainers, including two excellent dancers, a nightclub entertainment host, a troop of women singers, and even crooners, roped into performing on the Saturday night programs. The professional actors put on a weekly vaudeville show. The members of this group collected enough funds to handover to the purchasing committee, 100 Philippine pesos to purchase wood in order to build a platform. The camp carpenters did the work of constructing the movable platform, which was placed every Saturday night on the large patio in between the main buildings of the Santo Tomas University, with its grand Spanish architecture.

The main building consisted of large four-sided buildings, three stories high with long open galleries. It's large square courtyard between the four sides, known as the patio, was at all times an inactive center of campus life. On Saturday night, however, several thousand people assembled in the patio, sitting on the ground or armed with a camp chair or stool. The internees placed themselves in the center or in the corridor along the side of the buildings. The second- and third-floor windows made ideal box seats for the show. It was quite a sight to see the happy faces responding to the fun. Each Saturday night, the internees left with joy in their hearts and laughter echoing throughout the entire building.

The camp's kind electricians cleverly converted the old film milk cans into floodlights. Week by week, the performances became more and more professional and extravagant. It was difficult for the Japanese to understand how such enjoyment and hilarity could exist inside the internment camp. Many of the internees were homeless and had lost everything, yet, not only smiled but also laughed wholeheartedly. At the Saturday night show, the harsh reality we lived in disappeared within the crowded house of internees.

303

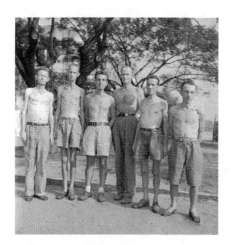

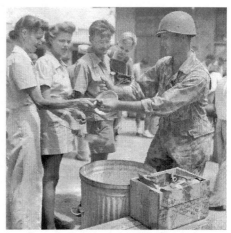

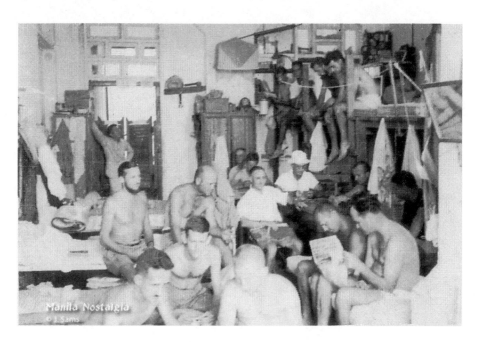

Internee life at Santo Tomas Internment Camp

Three Escapees

In February 1942, Singapore surrendered to the Japanese, and in March, the Dutch stronghold of Batavia on the island of Java surrendered. These two back-to-back losses signaled a turning point in the war, forcing Allied nationals to reconsider the strength of the Japanese navy and the prospects of an Allied victory in the East Asia sphere.

Three British internees, one of who had been second officer on the H.M.S. Anhwei, attempted to escape in March 1943 and were caught. They were found hiding among the jungles of the Ballantine peninsula. The three men received severe floggings. One of the guards who administered the beating came into the camp hospital later for treatment of a thumb that had been badly bitten by one of the prisoners during the flogging. A day or so later, the Japanese soldiers shot the three men. This event caused much indignation among the internees.

Many rumors spread among the internees following the men's arrest. They said the commandant took off his military uniform and went to the Japanese military headquarters in the city to plead for the lives of the three escapees. For whatever reason, it caused our camp commandant to be recalled shortly after the incident. The Japanese hired a disciplinarian commandant who replaced him. I believed they recalled him because he came to favor the internees too much.

In the early morning after the day of the shooting, a large crowd attended the funeral service, which was held in the Catholic chapel on the grounds of Santo Tomas. Internees from all faiths crowded in the chapel, surrounding the lobby and steps. All denominations of whatever faith or creed attended this mass for every person in his heart protested against the Japanese shooting the civilians.

A black cloud hovered over everyone at the camp for many days. The entertainers did not perform at our regular Saturday evening shows for weeks. No one had any heart for the light-hearted activities.

Captives of Empire: The Japanese Internment of Allied Civilians in China, 1941–1945

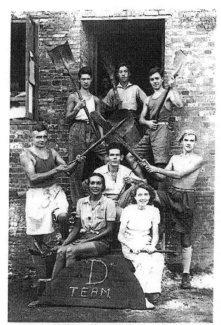

Kitchen team "D" at Yangchow C.

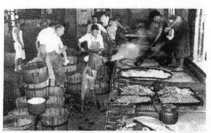

Lunghwa Camp kitchen.

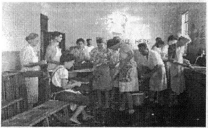

The scullery at Chapei.

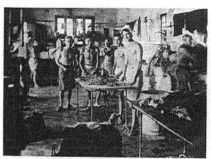

Kitchen crew at Stanley Camp.

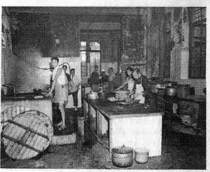

Yangtzepoo Camp kitchen.

The Triumphant Shacks in Santo Tomas

After six months of being held captive in the Santo Tomas Internment Camp, the Manila rainy season began in June. It lasted until October and was especially trying for us. At no time did any internee enjoy the muddy walks around the camp. In the dry season it had been dusty; in the rainy season, the grounds were so soupy and flooded in the low-lying areas that one had to wade through rivers and mush to go anywhere in the camp.

The hopelessness we felt during this time frustrated our spirits and tempers soared. The internees became even more disheartened when, on one very rainy day, a group of Japanese soldiers marched into our outdoor eating room area and, without a word to any of us, took down our prized circus tent—that had been protecting us from the penetrating heat of the sun while we ate at the covered tables—so we were now exposed to the downpour of rain. It felt as though they were pulling off our skin, as it was the one protection we had from the harsh heat and cold, rainy weather. For months, that tent had protected us in its arms and brought us together as one tribe under a safe shelter. We later heard that the Japanese did not care for our welfare and decided they needed it for their own purposes. So much of the internees' faith drowned in that act of c r u e l t y .

Day after day, we ate outdoors as the rain poured down on us and dampened our spirits. Many people grew angrier because there was no overhead shelter. It was one thing to have never had it, but to have had it and experienced the loss of it was far more devastating.

The pain of our loss turned into rage and some internees decided to rise to the occasion. It is true that when a demand becomes sufficiently great that ingenuity of man usually ascends to meet the occasion.

As a result of the loss of the protective circus tent, one person, followed by another, built little private shanties in the courtyard of the university campus—their own private huts, so they could share their meals and intimate time with their own family or friends. Within a few days, mini shelters popped up like mushrooms in a dark forest.

307

The first attempts were very crude. Branches of trees or pieces of wood picked up on the grounds sticking into the earth were propped up with string or wire. Old dilapidated bed quilts, torn sheets, table clothes, or pieces of torn sacking, which had been rescued from the discard, were stretched across the sticks to act as a sun breaker. They now seemed desperate to create something of their own.

How great the fall from the seeds of the mighty, millionaires who previously possessed a city home or country estate were reduced to living in homeless conditions that could well make the average city dweller smile in adoration. From one piece of line that connected the uprights also hung the washing, dishcloths towels, and clothing. Each person treasured their own possession of an enamel cup, bowl, and plate, with a knife, fork, and spoon, which constituted the tableware that they set on an old box used as a table for each mealtime.

After the first few months of building shanties, the efforts of the building committee made it possible to construct toilets, more showers, drains, and wash tubs. The committee permitted the purchase of sufficient wood to construct along an overhead shelter open at the sides. Wooden boards up on the trestles served as tables, and benches placed at the right angles on the roofing became sufficient to seat several hundred persons during meal times, twice daily.

At the end of the first year, around 4,500 internees and 600 individuals had built their own family shanties. The homes, however, were quite different from the pioneer's ragtag makeshift shacks that were first built after our beloved circus tent was taken away. The dwellings had wooden floors and *sawali*, or grass matting roofs. These up-to-date additions were being made possible because of the purchasing committee and the ingenuity of the campers vying with each other to see which could turn out the best shack with the most ingenious homemade gadgets.

308

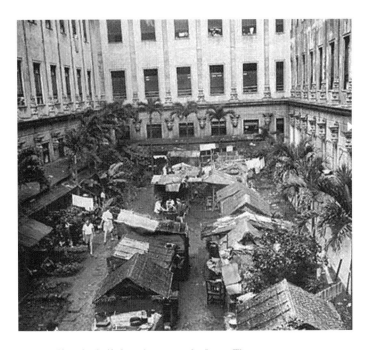

Shanties built by prisoners at the Santo Tomas camp

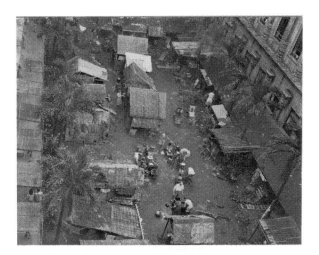

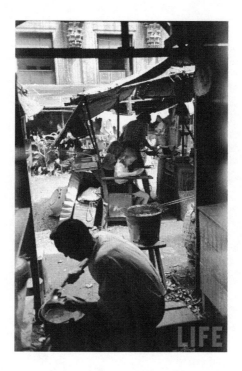

The shelters did provide a little overhead aid against the heat of the hot sun and wet, rainy season, but they provided a much greater reward. It gave the internees autonomy, inspiration, privacy, and hope for a better future. Each new house—each new idea they created a bigger, warmer, more efficient home for someone—gave each of us more faith that, in time, our lives would be better, safer, and possibly, easier.

Both sadly and triumphantly, on November 14, 1943, a typhoon dumped 27 inches of rain and wiped out most of the internees shanties. Despite the devastating conditions, the internees rebuilt their homes, and by Christmas, the Red Cross sent parcels for every person with food, medicine, and other supplies.

During this time, I made many great friends and was surrounded by good-hearted cheerleaders at the Santo Tomas Internment Camp. Major Colette, a fellow prisoner of war, became a dear friend of mine and told me often how I was an inspiration to her and other prisoners. Even during our hardships, I tried my best to endure our battle with a sense of humor and make it bearable, because there were others who were much far worse than me that needed our help.

Mrs. Martha Hill, a fellow prisoner who had been anaesthesiologist at the Sternberg Hospital, worked with me on patients. She often said I was a rock in a weary land and with a humorous sparkle in my eye. She thought I had good common sense, but would sometimes pour a little oil on the troubled waters. Even under these conditions, I still wanted others to like and respect me. I wanted to be a strong and stoic example to everyone else. I tried my best not to show my temper and become upset, not even when we waited in long terminal lines to get into the bathroom early in the morning, take a shower—with two others to conserve water—get food, and so on. I read my Bible every morning before I got up and often confessed to others that the day always seemed to go better for me when I read a psalm or two. The hymns the prisoners sang, "Great is Thy Faithfulness" and "When He Shall Come," were special favorites of mine.

Unbeknownst to me, my half-brother, William Edward Roberts, died on September 28, 1942 in Chicago, Cook County, Illinois, when I was 61 years old. I had not heard from my family for over a year. I had no doubt they were very worried; keeping my faith and saying daily prayers for them and all of the prisoners and Allied soldiers was a saving grace for me.

A Sad Occasion

Following the fall of Corregidor, General Jonathan Wainwright spoke over the local radio. The Japanese had forbidden radios in the camp, but a few engineers secretly salvaged parts from the commandant's radio and built their own. That's how we learned about Corregidor and learned that the tide of the war was turning against the Germans and Japanese. In April 1942, the first United States planes began flying over Manila on bombing runs. The internees would stand on the roof of the main university building and watch

311

Now the internees were listening to the United States Army broadcasted from Corregidor. The voice of freedom had been silent for almost two years. The last message I heard broadcast was on Easter Sunday, April 5, 1942. The announcer declared: we shall rise in the name of freedom and the East Shelby, a light with the glory of our liberation, and tell them people of the Philippines should be not afraid.

We kept the faith despite the next announcement on May 6, 1942, when General Wainwright had to announce to the different United States Army chiefs in the Philippine Islands that all firearms and ammunition must be turned over to the Japanese and that their complete surrender was obligatory. What a sad occasion indeed for an American general. For several hours previous to this surrender message, a local announcer requested that everyone listen for an important announcement. General Wainwright repeated his message four times, once to each of the four divisional army chiefs in the islands.

Those of us who listened to his words sunk into the internees' sense of desperation and wrung with sympathy for this man who was obliged to deliver this difficult and humiliating news, that Bataan and Corregidor who had gallantly defended their positions from December 8, 1941 to May 6, 1942 were now forced to surrender. The Japanese held General Wainwright and his command as prisoners of war for some months in the United States Army and Naval Club in Manila. He was later transferred to Formosa, along with the other Japanese prisoners of war.

The first year or so of encampment was difficult, but not as shocking as what was to come. As each week passed, each day we believed it would be over soon and America would save us, but as each week went by, we lost hope and became more uncertain and disheartened.

The last my family had heard from me was from the telegram I sent to them on December 22, 1941. It was not until the War Department sent an official letter to the Rockefeller Foundation that my family knew if I was alive or dead.

312

Thankfully, Lieutenant Colonel Howard F. Bresee wrote to them on behalf of the Office of the Provost Marshal General on August 3, 1943 that Miss Ethel Robinson, Dr. Frank E. Whitcare, and myself had been interned by Japan, but at the time, making the best of it. They directed them to send any correspondence to their office and the office would do their best to direct and guide it through the mail to us. Sadly, though, no mail was given to us, so for over a year and a half, my family had no idea what became of me.

Manila to Shanghai China

In the fall of 1942, I became ill with pneumonia. The hospital staff admitted me into the nurses' home in the Santo Tomas camp and Dr. Markusson oversaw my care. After a month, my condition worsened, and due to my age and the work at the Peiping Hospital in China, the doctors recommended that I be moved to Shanghai.

At the time, I felt very blessed to be given permission and my papers to take a boat to Shanghai in order to get the care I needed in a fully functioning hospital. While Shanghai was still under Japanese occupation, my hope was that I would be better cared for in nicer conditions than we had at our internment camp in Manila, and just possibly, get repatriation back to America.

This blessing would turn into a nightmare. I took a small tugboat from Manila via Wu Soong and transferred to a cattle boat. The boat carried destitute prisoners of war in the same container as the cattle. We slept on the floor for the duration. It pains me and turns my stomach inside out just writing about it. The boat ride from Manila to Shanghai took ten days and we all experienced unmitigated, excusable indignities and hardships at the hands of the Japanese.

I was shocked that I made the journey to Shanghai alive. Besides having experienced pneumonia for the last two months, I was very ill with beriberi, which was caused by my lack of nutrition and vitamin B1 deficiency, also known as thiamine deficiency. It affected my heart and circulatory system, and damaged my nerves, which led to my decreased muscle strength. This led me to experiencing polyneuritis.

313

It was a blessing that I had been warned before I left to carry a generous supply of peanut butter with me. Due to the deficiency, it was a miracle I did, as that peanut butter was the lifesaver I needed on the cattle boat from Manila to Shanghai.

My trip to Shanghai and the arrival was a "let down," to use a definite word, and actually, another tragic story I was determined to live to tell. We arrived at the dock with no assistance from anyone. Japanese soldiers barked orders and, dazedly, we had to find our way to the American Association headquarters of Swiss Consulate at 57 Canton Road. I stood in line waiting, trembling on my weak legs for hours. The church house was the headquarters for camp internees' information. I visited all three different buildings to get all of the necessary papers, signatures, etc.

By the time I checked in at Dr. Dunlap's home, where I was ordered to stay, I was so tired and went to bed for several days. Dr. Halpern, who examined me when I arrived, had been trying to get a bed for me in the county hospital. From his efforts, on January 22, he took me to the hospital and checked me in.

After recovering for six weeks of pneumonia, under the care of Dr. Josephine Lawney, MD, I was pronounced ready, or almost ready, to go to camp. Personally, it seemed to me that camp would by far be the safest place for me to be because pillaging was happening all over the city and my entire bedding roll was stolen from the recovery house the first day I was checked-in after I left the hospital.

Much uncertainty was likely. For example, possible coolie riots or Japanese repercussion on Americans out of the internee's camp helped me decide to try to carry on the rest of my time in China at camp. I felt I could conserve energy and perhaps be able to carry my own weight and be of some service in a quiet way.

In March, I finally found a way to send a telegram to my family. I addressed it to Archibald who lived at 46 Harrison Road in Brookline, Massachusetts. I wrote the following: "In hospital, health improved—left mail last September—hoping for repatriation—anxious to hear your news—much love, Mollie."

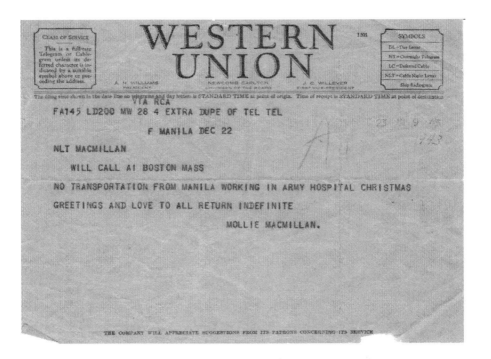

Telegram home to family after invasion and bombing of Manila

To The COMITE INTERNATIONAL DE LA CROIX-ROUGE
GENEVE (Suisse). SHANGHAI
Please transmit the following message:

DEMANDEUR — ANFRAGESTELLER — ENQUIRER

PLEASE WRITE IN BLOCK LETTERS.

Nom-Name... McMILLAN   Nationality... AMERICAN

Prénom-Christian Name-Vorname... MARY

Rue-Street-Strasse... c/o INTERNATIONAL RED CROSS

Localité-Locality-Ortschaft... SHANGHAI

Province-County-Provinz... KIANGSI

Pays-Country-Land... CHINA

AMERICAN RED CROSS
OCT 26 1943
INQUIRY UNIT

Message à transmettre—Mitteilung—Message
(25 mots au maximum, nouvelles de caractère strictement personnel et familial)—
(nicht über 25 Worte, nur persönliche Familiennachrichten)—(not over 25 words,
family news of strictly personal character).

IN HOSPITAL SHANGHAI HEALTH IMPROVED
LEFT MANILA LAST SEPTEMBER STILL
HOPING FOR REPATRIATION ANXIOUS TO
HEAR YOUR NEWS MUCH LOVE
MOLLIE

Date-Datum... MARCH 1943.

DESTINATAIRE — EMPFANGER — ADDRESSEE

PLEASE WRITE IN BLOCK LETTERS.

Nom-Name... McMILLAN   Nationality... AMERICAN

Prénom-Christian Name-Vorname... ARCHIBALD

Rue-Street-Strasse... 46 GARRISON ROAD

Localité-Locality-Ortschaft... BROOKLINE

Province-County-Provinz... MASSACHUSETTS

Pays-Country-Land... U.S.A.

ANTWORT UMSEITIG.   RÉPONSE AU VERSO   REPLY OVERLEAF
Bitte sehr deutlich schreiben!   Prière d'écrire très lisiblement!   Please write very clearly.

*International Red Cross cable to family while in hospital during internment
under Japanese occupation hospital*

JOSEPHINE C. LAWNEY, M. D.
11 MANOR AVENUE   ROSLYN HEIGHTS, LONG ISLAND, N. Y.

June 25, 1955.

To the War Claims Commission,
Washington, D. C.

Gentlemen:-

Miss Mary McMillan was my patient in a
Japanese Internment Camp in Chapel, Shanghai, China,
from February to September, 1943. She had made a
poor convalescence from pneumonia which she had contracted in Manila, had a marked polyneuritis and a
beri-beri heart from malnutrition. While she was
under treatment for these conditions, she suffered
a severe attack of herpes zoster of which we had
seven cases in camp in sequence from contacts.

Miss McMillan suffered worse permanent dis-
ability than any other of our one thousand internees
during the time I was in charge of the medical service.

Respectfully submitted,

Josephine L Lawney. M.D.

Chapei Japanese Internment Camp

The first week in April, I was driven by rickshaw with my little luggage to my new internment camp. I had heard it had the same basic setup as Santo Tomas, but it had better accommodations and food supplies.

When the Chapei Internment Camp first opened, the commandant, Riolo Tsurumi, and his assistant, Inaba, ran it. He greeted new arrivals with a speech intended to be both reassuring and threatening: "I, the Japanese Consul and the Commandant of this Civil Assembly Centre, give instruction to all to assemble here today. Unfortunately, the prevailing international circumstances have deprived you of your right to free life and necessitated to you to enter this place. However, this is your safest refuge where your rights are best guaranteed and the only abode you are now permitted to live in. You must, therefore, cope with the rules and regulations and make possible efforts in the carrying on of this place with a spirit of mutual harmony and with the thought that this is your home, loving it, enjoying your life and duties given to you. On this I emphasize. If contrary to the above, you should violate the regulations; you shall be punished according to the penal regulations. Should any of you attempt to run away from this place you might be shot to death by our guards. This you must remember. You must read, carefully, the regulations which are handed to you."

The Chapei Japanese Civil Assembly, located on Chungsan Road in northwest Shanghai, had already been captured in combat and the prisoners of war were relocated to Shanghai. The Chapei camp was predominantly made up of American and Dutch nationals. Their ages, occupations, and places of work were listed on their intake forms.

American families and unattached women had been notified a week or ten days ahead of time to report to the American Association, which was the "key" announcement known to mean but one thing: we were headed back into internment. And now I would be one of them.

I arrived and found the Chapei Internment Camp to be run very similar to the Santo Tomas camp. There was an executive board and different departments that took care of all the different internees needs. I did, however, notice that the American Red Cross was much more involved in the operation of this camp.

They served the meals at 7:00 a.m., which consisted of a breakfast cracked wheat, an American Red Cross contribution, with tea and eight ounces of dark bread for each person as their daily ration. Fried rice with greens and tea was set out at 11:00 a.m., in addition to some poor soup. The food was unappetizing and inadequate but not as bad as the other camp. The evening soup was our lunch, refurbished by adding Chinese shredded meat and catsup to make a type of stew. We sometimes added peanut butter and our own sugar, which we bought before camp, in allowance of three and a half ounces per month, per person, and jam or marshmallows, plus powdered milk. Occasionally, a tin of sausage and a vegetable was added to the meal to make a banquet.

We longed for fresh fruit, eggs, vegetables, more jam in liquid form, and a scant cereal allowance. What excitement it was when the first egg reached us, as we cackled about it all day. Occasionally, we get an apple; hundreds of people would stand in line and would be pleased as punch to get it.

Even though I was still very sick, they obliged each prisoner to serve at least three hours a day, and many, such as office workers, served eight or more hours. Cooks worked in shifts, a regular squad of all women—except those engaged in a hospital or office— scraped, paired, and cleaned every day in the kitchen. The weather was very hot and the assignees started at 5:30 a.m., which I found difficult to wake up for.

Squads worked daily in debugging cracked wheat and rice, a tedious and difficult job. Rice was all we ate until comfort money came in the middle of May. The greens purchased were hard to clean; in fact, the whole really only fit for garbage, yet the Japanese complained of cleaning so we had to instead.

319

Because almost everything in a way of food, tea, coffee, and drinks had   to be purchased, the amount was quite inadequate on account of crowded conditions, which were comprised of bunks twenty inches wide grouped and 240 women slept in these bunks in one section of the deck.

A bathhouse with ample hot and cold showers had been erected by internees and later, three tubs with faucets for washing clothes. It was a great blessing indeed. Washing laundry was a daily task. We washed sheets and bed linens manually until later a laundry opened, but things came back badly torn and with bad colors so after many had the washing habit, it seemed to stick.

Not until the middle of May did our blessings fall one upon the other; the opening of the camp canteen and the United States comfort money. The comfort money was distributed for camp internees' food supplies. They were given an amount of 300 or 400 yen per month for the chef to buy vegetables, carrots, onions, occasionally white potatoes, and quite often, sweet potatoes, an egg per person each day, and a small amount of powdered milk.

In the beginning of summer the internees became overwhelmed by receiving an apple or pear almost once a week and with an egg a day, we strutted like lords. Each person was assigned so much peanut butter for a month—half a pound, and one pound of sugar, one or two biscuit packs, and a treat with raspberry jam. A few weeks later, they added canned salmon.

Floors were assigned to internees later as the line-ups of well-nigh 1,000 persons standing for hours in the sun were not only time-consuming and exhausting, but several persons fainted, and others had bad heart spells. The demand for canteen goods continued, although the long lines continued. The hours of purchase were limited and not open every day; only when supplies arrived.

The education committee, headed by Dr. Mae Muller of Nanking, had planned a fine education program. The students found it difficult to acquire sitting space in a shed and labored vehemently under adverse conditions for supplies and space. The regular school curriculum was carried as though as in Manila.

320

After three months, unfortunately while I was under treatment for my health conditions, I suffered a severe attack of herpes zoster, of which they had seven cases in the camp in sequence from contacts. Dr. Lawney shook her head when she diagnosed me and said she believed I had suffered worse health than over 1,000 internees she had seen during this period of time.

The camp infirmary had about twenty beds and a busy daily clinic at which a well-balanced group of doctors and specialists took care of our needs. Nurses were scarce, so nursing aides were trained and took duty daily on schedule, as did the registered nurses. They assigned two night nurses per shift, and for any serious illnesses like pneumonia, specialists were at hand.

An epidemic of whooping cough caused such disruption to nursing staff, a room to hold 50 or so was given over to the "whoopers," and quite a few cases of measles. Then an epidemic of intestinal trouble fell upon the camp in June and hit 700 out of 1,000 internees hard. A definite bacillus was not found in lab findings. It had been spoken of as a nutritional diarrhea from some tainted meat and molded bread due to extremely inadequate refrigeration. Therefore, it was no surprise that gastrointestinal disturbances were all over the camps.

The most serious cases and operations the doctors sent out to hospital and each case personally had to be brought to the Japanese Commandant by the chief doctor before permission was granted.

Weekly reports from the hospital superintendent about the patient's condition had to be submitted, noting when recovery was sufficient to return to camp.

A car took patients to and from and made a charge of several hundred dollars each way for a trip. All money had to be given as soon as internees entered camp, letters of credit, checks, gold, etc. The Mitsubishi Bank had the cash, and we were given bank books, but we were only allowed to spend at the canteen by purchasing goods that were to be put on account against our account for exchange of money. Before leaving, they gave us the balance of our account up to the sum of $5,000 CRB and were told that $500 or $600 was all we needed on the trip.

The large main camp shed was where the school classes, dining room, a meeting place for lectures every evening, concert hall, and a church were held. Catholic early services were held every day with two priests only. All Protestant and other church denominations worshiped together. They conducted church services in sheds and early dining rooms had to be given up for later internees as the shed was the only place in stormy or rainy weather, it was not at all a desirable place being entirely open to the elements; consequently most people ate in their own rooms. This meant walking up and down four flights of stone and two floors, then down again for a hot dish, water, and garbage three times a day.

Bishop Roberts who worked on the kitchen squad and sang in the choral choir of all denominations also conducted some services, along with Dr. Slavly Smith of the Church of Shanghai. They were largely responsible for excellent cooperation of all worshiping groups.

The library in Chapei had extremely good books from an American school and from the Shanghai City Club with many personal donations that so little was left to be desired. Professional librarians filed books and conducted loans as in public libraries. Pre-nursery schools enabled parent's time for play and reading. One of the most tedious daily tasks was standing in a queue, especially folks with youngsters, as children in food lines were earlier than either the second or first calls and were anxious to eat.

Sports did not take quite the same place in Chapei as they did in Manila for adults owing to more limited quarters; most of the place was not designed for school-age children. Almost every afternoon though, a school baseball and English cricket game was played with quite an audience of parents and those interested.

They planned amusements and informal evening jams with piano accompaniment: Ed Mackay as leader; James Dunlap, violin; Dr. Hugh Walters and Mr. Deitch as guitarists; banjoist; and Janice as a professional cellist. Excellent musicians, who led music, when required, later augmented this group; they also had most of this group for Sunday high mass and evening song.

Gaul's Holy City presented four soloists and capable efficient Myra Olive as chorus and choir leader. An excellent concert or two, good church choir music were the outstanding features of Myra Olive's valuable service to the camp. A couple of variety shows owe their greatest credit to Billy and Carol who labored untiringly and were capable of arranging very excellent programs. They had cheetahs dancing; professional and exquisite, her cleverness and ability at writing words and sonnets had full play.

On July 4, 1943, the camp was filled with hope, joy, and celebration that we would soon be rescued. We signed our release papers in Chapei Internment Camp and waited to board the first repatriation ship that was to sail in September.

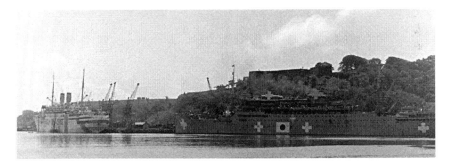

The Teia Maru ship (above) sailing American internees to be exchanged for Japanese civilians prior to boarding the Gripsholm ship (top) in 1943. The 1943 repatriation voyage was one of the most significant for both ships and well-documented. This photo shows the two ships lined up at the dock in Mormugao.

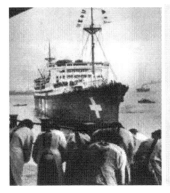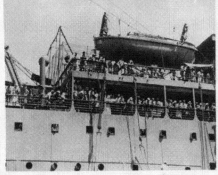

Teia Maru

Approximately 1,000 of us Chapei internees nervously boarded the Teia Maru ship on September 19, 1943 at Whangpao. The ship flew the Japanese flag but originally flew the French flag and was named the MS Aramais. The passenger ship had been seized by Japan in 1942.

When we boarded the ship, we met 80 or so American repatriates who came from Japan. We crammed into the already packed ship, which had not been well taken care of. They assigned our cabins varying from first, second, or third class located on the upper decks; the steerage area, considered the lower class area, consisted of wooden bunks and a straw mattress with a sheet, blanket, and pillow.

They designed the ship to accommodate 800 passengers, but after the Japanese took it over, they added wooden bunks everywhere they could to squeeze even more on and put beds on the promenade deck.

I was lucky that priority was given to the aged women, children, and sick. We were given the best classes, and the strongest middle-aged men given the lower class. I shared a comfortable room with a sound mattress, wardrobe, and bathroom. The room was nothing compared to my room on the Empress of Japan, but a happy change from where I had laid my head for the last three years.

The nursery on deck bunked an additional four-dozen women. The bunks were two-decked, with narrow awareness between rows. Many of these women were obliged to use bathrooms on lower floors, owing to great water shortages and lack of bathrooms. Even daily bathing was impossible except in cabins where there was a basin. Those of us fortunate enough to have a basin had a regular daily time and for those lacking, we shared with friends to come in and do their daily personal bathing and washing. After the first week, no laundry was taken on the ship.

324

I was even obliged to wash my own sheets in deference to cleanliness. Part of the deck looked like a backyard on washday with community scale washing.

Each class ate in their own dining rooms, but was served the same dire food. Breakfast was rice porridge and sometimes a little scrambled eggs with boiled potatoes. Lunch was soup, bread, vegetables, and gelatin; and dinner was rice, curry, fruit, or cake. They served us decent but small portions of food. I am not sure the passengers on the lower decks fared as well.

I ate in first class and fared better than many of my friends and neighbors, but it meant arriving at 6:00 a.m. or thereabouts to be on hand for 7:00 a.m. breakfast and 4:00 p.m. for the evening meal at 5:00 p.m. The scanty food and butter pads on each plate became smaller and smaller, as well as bread, tea, and coffee (only a quarter, or at most a third, filled a cup already sweetened with a bare coloring of milk). For extra money, they sold tea, coffee, bread, butter, and cheese. They even charged passengers for a thermos filled with hot water. The food sold helped to keep up moderate diet and necessities, which meant giving lots of gratuities to the Japanese steward.

The dishwasher only wiped off the plates, cups, and glasses with no attempt to washing. No table napkins or towels were provided. Our sheets, pillowcases, and table clothes were changed once in 30 days. They rarely cleaned the cabins and most of the time did not clean at all. Never have I seen such a dirty ship, disgustingly so, and short on stewards.

We sailed again on September 20, arrived in Hong Kong on September 23, picking up another 24 prisoners of war at the anchorage off Stanley Prison. We pulled up to the island on the Stanley side, not on the Kowborn as planned. The island was very beautiful and the Stanley Internment Camp seemed to certainly have the advantages of a beautiful location.

325

Sixty-three internees came aboard and looked happy and relieved to finally be rescued. We began to worry about the additional stops and more passengers boarding, as lack of food when we arrived at Hong Kong was a serious problem. If something was not forthcoming from this port, the doctors told us that illness and other serious complications might arise, which could be incurable because of our   food spoiling due to the lack of proper storage.

It was poisoning us. I never learned if, or how much, food was loaded on the ship after Hong Kong but we stayed in port for 30 hours.

One of the people who boarded was Father Murphy, a young 30-year-old priest and a Canadian Catholic who studied at the Maryknoll House in Hong Kong at the outbreak of hostilities. He carried a very great responsibility regarding the welfare of material as well as of spiritual things. There were about 60 priests and 90 nuns on board, and each evening at sunset, they faced toward the evening star and chanted in harmony the song of prayer and protection to the star of the sea.

During the song, I saw Father Murphy's whole frame shake and tears roll down his face. One could imagine what the feeling of safety was for the people leaving in hope of spreading prayers and enough hope to get the others released. It does not take a great imagination to realize what it meant to an earnest and devoted Christian that this prayer was a song for protection.

The next day, we sailed to San Fernando, La Union, Philippines, and 130 more passengers boarded. Repatriates from camps at Santo Tomas, Los Banos, and Baguio had arrived by train and boarded. Out of the 100 repatriates, there were 60 Catholic priests—Americans, Canadians, and a few Spanish—and eight nuns. Also present were Protestant missionaries with a handful of men, women, and children. The passengers grew weary and hungrier with each stop. We hoped the end of the journey would come soon and yearned for our freedom.

We sailed by pilot up to Mekong River to within sites of Saigon. The trip down the river offered the passengers outstanding features and a most unusual experience. We spoke about how we were prisoners of war traveling over 20,000 miles around the world as a repatriate. What great stories we would have to share when we returned home.

Our ship was winding down the river, in and out of narrow spots and wide at others, jungle on either side with dense foliage and small native mud pots at intervals of a mile. The mystic haze that accompanied the glowing sunsets were seen so frequently near the equator where the sun disappeared; a breathtaking, gorgeous splendor within a very short period. We saw one of the most extravagant peaks as we sailed down the Mekong River in twilight. Tropical foliage and jungle colors and native settings were bewitching, and we were gloried in God's masterpiece.

We sailed into the Pacific Ocean due south to Singapore and waited outside Singapore for two days to take on water. About 30 more prisoners boarded on the October 5. A few of them were high-level executives, with National and Chase Bank, in addition to a British-American tobacco company. After leaving Singapore, we prayed for a better water supply, but no improvement occurred. We only had water for two hours daily, and sometimes, not even that.

We sailed to Goa following south passageway through the Sunda Strait, and not north using the Strait of Malacca. We sailed along the east coast of Sanabria between Sumatra and Java with Bornia near the east, to the southern tip of India, then up a few hundred miles to Portuguese India and the island of Goa. Calm seas cooled and calmed the passengers for the last ten days of our journey as we crossed the equator—twice—on the near east side of Singapore and west side of Sumatra.

We had high hopes that our boat would soon meet of the MS Gripsholm in Mormugao in Portuguese India, a small coastal enclave near Goa that was neutral Portuguese territory surrounded by the British India Empire.

327

Our Japanese naval transport, Teia Maru, carried 1,500 Western Hemisphere nationals interned in the Orient that were to be exchanged for the 1,330 Japanese civilians aboard the liner MS Gripsholm.

After almost a month, we finally arrived in the port of Mormugao in Goa, on October 17, at noon. A beautiful, lush, green scene with trees and an old stone fort was our first view. We stood, crowded on the decks, and watched as our luggage was moved from the ship's cargo area by crane to the shore and carried by Indian porters to another area for unpacking and repacking. Newspaper correspondents met the ship to get pictures and interviews with the United States internees.

The next day the Teia Maru, repatriates split into four groups in alphabetical order and were allowed to step on shore to line up

at sheds to get passes, check our luggage, and get warmer clothes for the next part of our journey, as it would be cold. They told us to return to the ship within one hour and we were only to go near sheds during our period ashore.

We had heard from the young American Maritime's service lads serving their first assignment with the United States government that we would receive good food on the MS Gripsholm. Most of the American children had sampled some food when the stewards and American lads brought sacks full of candy bars and ice cream on the wharf for children. There was a mad rush to snatch food, of course, because they had been suffering for good food, not only for the last four weeks on the Teia Maru, but for more than two years as Manila and Hong Kong internees. With great anticipation, the MS Gripsholm pulled into the wharf on Saturday the eighteenth.

The boat was quite a contrast to the ugly gray Japanese Teia Maru, where the Japanese flag was hung from the mast.

328

The MS Gripsholm was painted white with the name of the vessel across top outside, MS Gripsholm Sverige and Diplomat painted in the area, and the Swedish flag and the words "Gripsholm Sverige and Diplomat" prominently on the whole side of the ship.

The Japanese aboard sang their national war song and stewards under the boat waved a reply from the stern. Then at last, they took down their flag, folded it, and all of the passengers cheered. We remained aboard their respective ships until the formalities of the exchange had been worked out. Finally, on Tuesday, October 19, after four days in port, hot nights, and spending a month on a dirty ship with poor conditions and scant food, in addition to a shortage of water, we were about to be freed.

The exchange of internees took place on the morning, an excellently planned affair after breakfast. All of us stood by our cabins. All baggage, except for our nightclothes, had been collected the previous evening and put on board the MS Gripsholm, along with Japanese baggage placed on their ship.

The internees lined up; a one-to-one for the exchange took place. I took a long deep breath in anticipation of the momentous transaction. Our freedom was so close and getting home to those I loved was now only a month away.

At 9:00 a.m., approximately 1,500 of Teia Maru's passengers lined up, except for a few stretcher cases, and within one hour's time, the deck was cleared from the lowest to the highest deck. The rescued prisoners walked in a queue from the gangway of the Teia Maru to the gangway on MS Gripsholm.

One by one, one Japanese left the MS Gripsholm and stepped aboard the Teia Maru, then one American stepped off the Teia Maru and boarded the MS Gripsholm by way of another gangway. There was a constant stream of moving internees for over an hour, one person moving one way and the other moving the opposite way. Never to be forgotten for all of the prisoners was the first buffet luncheon on the MS Gripsholm.

329

We were delighted over tables that had a smorgasbord of bread, beef, turkey, ham, cheese, vegetable salad, hard-boiled eggs, cucumbers, pickles, olives, stewed fruits, and iced tea with lemon. It was hard not to overeat and we had been warned we

could get very sick if we ate too much because of our malnourishment. Never had food been better appreciated than to the half-starving internee passengers. We ate with tears of joy and savored every bite.

They handed out vitamin packs to help build up our deficiencies again. The Red Cross also distributed warm clothing, underwear, sweaters, and socks to the destitute internees who had been wearing the same clothes—in some cases, for two years.

Many of us became overwhelmed and tears flowed when bundles of mail from our friends and families were set out on tables and handed out in alphabetical order (news of whether husbands were alive or dead, birth announcements, and people still missing in combat).

On board the MS Gripsholm, we had about 63 nurses, 42 doctors, and a couple dozen nurses who belonged to mission groups in China, Japan, and French Indochina. The Chilean ambassador's wife from Tokyo was aboard and around 25 others in the diplomatic group. Most of this group kept quite busy with the internee's affairs.

Two copies of long, four-page questionnaires were handed out to all of the repatriates to fill out. Other papers from the maritime commission and questionnaires on personal dealings with the Japanese were gathered and recorded. Consequently, "Uncle Sam" had hired many of the internees for typing. The United States government set up a large room on the MS Gripsholm and filled it with typewriters for that purpose.

That evening on the promenade deck, the happy repatriates sat under colored awning at tables in elegant chairs quite different from the ones on the Teia Maru.

It looked like a swimming pool area of a European spa. The internees' faces, one weary, assumed a joyous looks, and some passengers burst out into song, "God be with you until we meet again."

For the first few hours, there was laughter and gaiety among all, a regular metamorphosis of humanity. The Red Cross handed out chocolate and cigarettes. They offered us food, drink, and hospitality without us asking as we waited for our rooms to be cleaned and assigned.

There were over 500 very nice cabins that accommodated two to four people. When the stewards began calling out our names and cabin numbers, it looked like Grand Central Station in New York as everyone scuttled to find their cabins. The MS Gripsholm stayed in Goa's port for twelve days, but it did not matter because we were all free.

The first day on the water was smooth but the next morning it became choppy, and the third and fourth days got worse. Both fortunately and unfortunately, the ex-internees had eaten so much after being starved for the last three years that one could see and hear passengers running in and out of the bathrooms due to seasickness.

Port Elizabeth, South Africa

Our entire trip had been very pleasurable and restful, although one elderly man, who had several earlier strokes, passed away. A minister or two were allowed on shore for the burial services where the deceased was buried on the slopes of a beautiful little Episcopal church on the hill. The wife and children of Mr. Arthur lived in America. One other death of a very sick man occurred aboard the MS Gripsholm. His body was buried at sea, and his widow, Mrs. Turner, stayed on board. There were also two suicides: one Japanese who drowned and one steward while inbound aboard the MS Gripsholm.

Twelve more days going south and again crossing the equator brought us to the tip of South Africa, and we landed in Port Elizabeth before noon on November 3. What a kind welcome awaited us on arrival, with buses to carry us to Featherstone Hull! On November 2, we anchored in Port Elizabeth, South Africa.

The next morning we ate breakfast and they told us we could visit the city to get our money from promissory notes for South African currency, get our land permits, and shop. Many of the citizens wanted to meet and host the passengers at their homes. Mrs. R. Searle, a British woman, pulled up and took Rand and me by car to their lovely home four miles out, where a home luncheon had been laid out. They wanted us to be their entire guests for two days, but we declined and left that afternoon for the city.

Dorothy St. Clair, of the Peiping Embassy, had traveled two nights and one day on a train from Pretoria to meet us. She appeared in my cabin before I was out of bed the next day and invited me to attend the mayor's party, given in our honor, for the internees, from 4:00 p.m. to 6:00 p.m. at the city hall. I had to pinch myself several times to believe all of this enjoyment was real.

We enjoyed the delightful party; the mayor and Rotary Club provided tables of food and drinks, as well as one or two short welcome addresses, with replies. A band played and many danced at the gay festivities. I became tired enough to return to the ship in time for supper and to be picked up by a private motor and brought to the gangplank by a man from Lancashire, England, who was a resident in Port Elizabeth.

Soon after 8:00 a.m. the following day, Rand and I started out by streetcar to the Homewood area, a drive along the shorefront to Happy Valley. It was a natural cliff between two hills with a well- wooded natural setting, much embellished by formal flower beds and walks, lotus ponds, stone bridges, and more—not at all spoiled by man's intervention.

We walked for about half a mile into the valley and it was well worthwhile. We returned in time to join Dorothy's party lunch at Cleghorne, the chief department store where good food was served. Then we looked around shops, bought a few Christmas cards, and returned to the ship. Our ship had been scheduled for us to leave by 4:00 p.m., but was delayed a couple of hours due to late-arriving passengers and crew, several of the latter who were so drunk they had to be dragged aboard.

For a few days, the ship slowed down to a crawl at certain places. We heard that there might be mines and our good captain was protecting us. We reached Rio de Janeiro early on November 15 due to heavy fog over the city. The captain felt obliged to wait until the fog lifted during this time, from 9:00 a.m. to noon, and we had the opportunity of observing one of the most beautiful harbors in the world.

Rio lies at the foot of mountain ranges, all of which are several hundred feet above sea level. Suburban houses were on mountainsides, all red-roofed, and the great new business buildings and apartment houses looked as white and clean as marble along the waterfront.

Above the city, situated on the peak of Mount Corvcoado, stood an inspiring sentinel, the most impressive white stone figure of Christ standing with outstretched arms. It stood over 100 feet high and is known as "Christ the Redeemer." The statue holds out his arms as if he is welcoming and protecting the whole city. When you gaze at it from out at sea, it looks like a white cross, and then when you get closer you can see that it almost seems like the statue is alive and offering you a warm invitation. At night, it is flooded in grace by searchlights. The ship made a stop in Rio de Janeiro, Brazil on November 16, and they told us we could leave the ship. This adventure would be our first taste of freedom.

We had luncheon aboard the ship and formed long, drawn out lines on the lower deck to visit the city. Miss Hodgman was there to greet us with open arms and her great loving heart, ready to pour out all she was able to in kindness and happiness.

333

We had a lovely bundle of mail, among which was a letter from Gertrude, offering a bed at her hotel overnight and a card of invitations to a buffet supper. Rand and I took a car around the city to view the beautiful botanical gardens, the Sugarloaf Mountain, and across the peak on the suspension car from which a magnificent view of the city, ocean, and shoreline were also visible.

We went back to Port Hotel, washed, and arrived at the buffet supper on a veranda with provisions made for 60 guests. Many of our North China friends were invited, and such a spread of cold turkey, dressing, many salads, prepared fruits, orange aide, demitasse, and chocolates preceded cocktails. It was a great feast, befitting the grand view of the harbor with all of its twinkling lights along the promenade—a sight never to be forgotten. My heart felt overjoyed as I thought about the last three years of deprivation and the happiness of the future.

The following day we walked around to shops with our hostess and saw the office of our friend working for the Institute of International Asian Affairs. We also visited Corcovado and got up close to view Christ with his outstretched arms, a stunning view where we could see part of the harbor and city.

Finally, we forced ourselves back aboard the ship around 9:00 p.m. We retired to our cabins, washed up, and ate supper, dead tired because we spent the day out and about from 8:00 a.m. to 9:00 p.m. Our North China friends greeted us with joy because it was something we had dreamed of for over two years.

In comparing notes from other camps while on the MS Gripsholm, each of the prisoners had their sad tragic stories to share. Locations, climate, crowded conditions, commandants' reactions—all "nuts to crack" for the executive committee. Many of the executives worked harder in the camp than in their own private or public enterprises in normal times. Working hard with the inadequate food supply or balanced diet was largely accountable for a sudden drop in weight in Manila, and the horrific conditions were an unexpected onslaught and a big psychological factor in the struggle for survival.

No prisoner I talked to, not even the regular residents in Manila ever expected a war as imminent and felt it might not come for months, if at all. The Japanese called their bluff, and we fell for it. The Chapei transients had at least a week or two of expectations going into camp so they could prepare—to some extent—food, clothing, and medical supplies, and were able to carry in bed and bedding and get cash by the United States government loan through the Swiss consul to purchase things. This option was not possible in Manila. Residents there did not get so many things from these loans, but as transients, we had neither funds nor cash. In all camps, a low-calorie food count was evident in the food provided by the Japanese.

They estimated that we had all eaten well under 1,000 calories daily and some as low as 600, so supplementing food was a necessity to sustain life. Even life of a sedentary nature, 2,400 calories was considered a necessary daily amount. Balance a diet with too much in carbohydrates, too little in fat and sugars, and no fruits with insufficient proteins and lack of calcium, along with vitamins and ascorbic acid, led to ripe conditions of severe malnutrition and disease. And sadly these illnesses went on for three years or more for some.

Both in Manila and Shanghai camps, persons suspected of being able to reveal information to the Japanese were placed into the prisoner camp, like Belabid in Manila or Bridge House in Shanghai. In Manila, several patients returned or came into camp from Belabid to forms of treatment to extract information. They would bind their thumbs on both hands so tightly that within a few hours, a prisoner was forced to talk, and if he didn't, a total paralysis resulted, a heavy stick inserted between both elbows.

One patient had a total paralysis of both hands as a result, another had partial paralysis that slowly improved with physical therapy treatments. A man over 60 years old, whose only suspect was that a young man came here to Manila with air troops, was told he was suspected of knowing where military stores were kept. They tortured him daily to extract information.

When his arms improved, the man was sent out to Philippine General Hospital for several weeks. Good food, rest, and care did wonders.

Manila was 50 acres wide and only three feet above sea level. Malaria and dengue fever spread quickly; a total loss of weight per person for the first year was around 30 pounds.

The internees' weight decreased owing to a shortage of food, becoming very serious in Manila and Hong Kong. The latter suffered even more that Manila; as an island cut off from mainland supplies, signs of possible blindness were getting much too common, owing to a shortage of citrus fruits, especially rich in vitamin C and ascorbic acid. In Haifeng Road, mostly political prisoners loss weight, an average of twenty pounds; Chapei averaged a loss of weight of 25 pounds.

Both Dr. Dave HFR and Dr. HK Graves spoke of reduced blood pressure as help in some cases of former highs. In Manila, there were a few isolated cases of measles; and chicken pox in Chapei, along with a big epidemic of whooping cough and quite a few measles. These children's epidemics made it very difficult to run an infirmary; isolation in very limited hospital quarters necessitated the commandeering of many of the parents' services as much as possible for day and night duty. As nurses and aides had a full-time schedule before the epidemic—not less than four to five hours daily duty and no personal laundry—cleaning of floor space and bedding was necessary in order to live. Standing in a queue for meals and washing took up much time, making the days full, overflowing in many instances, leaving everyone so physically worn out, that a bed was very welcome.

The story of the noble and heroic efforts of our brave men will go down in history. The loss of life was heavy, and the suffering of the men who were taken as prisoners by the Japanese has all been graphically told. For those who were fortunate enough to escape, the memory of those days were severed into their hearts like coals of fire—this memory of their comrades.

A few hours after Pearl Harbor, the Japanese captured a United States Army post; within a couple of days they had Cavite Navy Yard, and a week or so later Japanese troops, in great numbers, had ended in Lingayen Gulf north of Manila and swept up everything as they advanced.

Within the first week, practically all American restorative possibilities had been exhausted. It was not much use having the front door barred and bolted if the back door was wide open; corridor still stands, but what a futile effort to fight, inevitably, a losing game. Our troops were inadequately armed and equipped, with an appalling shortage of aircraft and no help to come as had been promised.

Away we sailed from Rio, this time from Pacific to Atlantic westward, to home and our loved ones. The ship was at times calm, and other times choppy, on the high seas. On the long homeward journey to New York, the captain steered out into the mid-Atlantic to avoid German submarines, which were active along the coast. One day, our ship passed a burning ship that had just been torpedoed, but was directed to pass by it without assisting. An undercurrent of nervousness filled the passengers' emotions on the boat for fear that the Germans were near.

On December 1, 1943, the MS Gripsholm finally entered the harbor and the sight of the landmarks of New York caused the passengers to cry tears of joy and shout out loud, "Oh my, there's the Statue of Liberty." We finally entered the harbor of our beloved New York, and it was with great joy that the county welcomed us as the MS Gripsholm sailed into the port. We were home at last. Dorothea Beck, the editor of the *Physical Therapy Review*, met me at the boat and hugged me with a great love and compassion I so needed to feel. For the first time in over three years, I took a deep breath and cried for all of the hardships endured, as well as the enriching experiences.

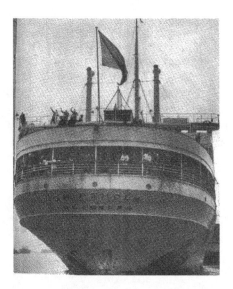

FRIENDS AND KIN CONVERGE ON N.Y. TO MEET GRIPSHOLM REPATRIATES

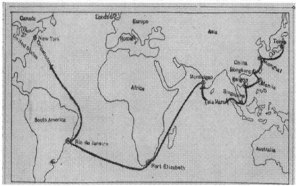

Desperation and
Ruthlessness Continues

In February 1944, the Americans continued to fight and make gains. The more the Allies fought, the more the Japanese became angrier at our country and the internees. As Japanese resources dwindled, they decided to move the Baguio internees to Manila because they expected MacArthur and his men to take back the Lingayen Gulf.

The longer the prisoners stayed in their internment camp, the worse the conditions became. At a certain point in 1944, the Japanese became ruthless and took over running the camp and food distribution. Their fortunes had turned against them, therefore the health and well being of the internees became less important. They cut off all contact with the outside world. Once they began to handle the food supply, people were dying of malnutrition and starvation by the end of the year. Their anger became unbearable and civilians were beaten just for not bowing correctly to them, but by far, the worst part was the agonizing hunger they felt every day. The food became less available to the internees, and they ate insects and plants from the gardens they had planted. At one point, the guards told them it was illegal to pick the greens and would not allow any outside help from charities.

On September 21, 1944, the United States Navy sent their bombers, and forces moved in closer to Manila. This mission was the first sign of hope that the internees had after almost three years as prisoners. Then, on October 20, they invaded the Philippines island of Leyte. Imagine the joy of the American prisoners of war and the thousands of internees at Santo Tomas when it was broadcast that there were good tidings of the landing of American troops on the island of Leyte.

The United States Army broadcasting station from Corregidor, the voice of freedom, had been silent for almost three years. The last message broadcast was on Easter Sunday 1942, which announced: we shall rewrite in the name of freedom and alight with the glory of our liberation and tell the people of the Philippines not to be afraid.

In October 1944, think of the rapture these words conveyed to thousands of war weary Americans and Philippines. The day of deliverance was at hand—this was the voice of freedom as General MacArthur was speaking.

Life conditions, starvations, and fear grew rampant around the Santo Tomas camp after this because the Americans began another daily round of Manila bombing, with low-range fighter planes. The Japanese's unrest had grown more desperate, and they killed 150 United States prisoners of war; some internees believed they would be next.

My friends there told me that on that day, there was a buzz in the air around camp that MacArthur and his forces would finally rescue the internees, but they feared that the Japanese would kill them before they would let that happen. Many internees said, "If I can only hold on for a little while longer, they will be here," but on January 9, 1945, the Japanese fought off the American troops again.

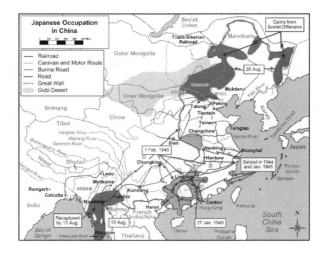

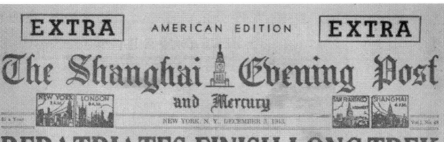

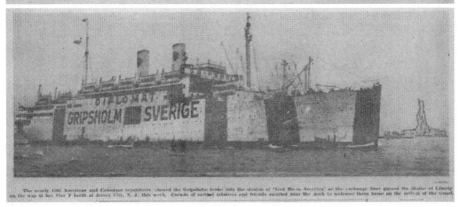

The Shanghai Evening Post American Edition, Dec. 3, 1943, page 1.

Credit to MRL 12: Foreign Missions Conference of North America Records, Series 2B, Box 33, Folder 9,

The Burke Library Archives (Columbia University Libraries) at Union Theological Seminary, New York.

15

FREEDOM

A fter I returned home, there would still be a few more months of heartache for me as I felt helpless over the 4,000 prisoners who were still in the Santo Tomas Internment Camp. Even though we experienced beriberi, edema, nerve damage, starvation, and death, we became a strong but weary tribe, and built our own city out of the ruins of an unjust and cruel war. Despite our difficult communal life, however, one did feel the full depth of daily living: kind services by our comrades willingly rendered, without money or without price; those kind deeds accepted gratefully and appreciatively, carried one far from the work-a-day world where each person may be out to get all they can.

Living as we did, material things lost their value; new subtle values, nevertheless real, arose in their stead. We had experienced a warm benevolent glow of friendship in spite of our difficult living conditions and lack of freedom. In this atmosphere, one found not only the strength of living, but also was given glimpses of God's grace and the best of the human race.

I was one of the few lucky prisoners of war, due to my brother's management of my finances. I was surprised to find out I was considered quite "wealthy" for that time in history. For me, after all those years of working, I lived comfortably, but not lavishly, for after all, I was a "Scot"—but my money could not heal my ill health or worry about my fellow prisoners who were still suffering.

The Japanese knew they had to delay the Americans for as long as possible, then they would have more time to prepare their own country for invasion. MacArthur told the United States that he had intercepted a message from Tokyo that General Yamashita was planning on executing all of the Allied prisoners and internees in the Cabanatuan and Santo Tomas camps before they were liberated. He directed General Mudge, and the 1st Cavalry Division, to begin moving into Manila to save and protect them.

I read the daily newspapers and wrote letters back and forth to anyone who might offer me information about my fellow prisoners. On January 30, the 6th Ranger Battalion rescued over 500 prisoners of war in Cabanatuan who had been too weak to be sent to labor camps. Then on February 1, American air fleet and tank troops broke though the Japanese lines into Manila.

I later heard from my friends in the camp that after they returned home on February 3, 1945, it was like any other day. The bombings continued and the prisoners stood in line to go to the bathroom, take a shower, and again stand in a long line for breakfast at 6:00 a.m. The internees were hesitant to look up because they had been told by the Japanese to never look up at the planes or they would be beaten.

They went about their daily chores that day, but the energy was different. They smelled fear in the air, not our fear but the Japanese in camp who had retreated into the men's building. Very few were on the site. They looked up and heard the sound of American aircraft engines getting closer and closer, flying lower and lower.

From an open bomber plane, one officer attached a note to his goggles and threw it into the courtyard. It read, "Roll out the barrels, for the gang's all here," which was a popular American polka theme song. Word spread around camp that our forces were finally coming to save the prisoners and the end was near. This message, that eventually reached over 4,000 exhausted and bedraggled internees at Santo Tomas camp, did not fail to help spring them to life when they recognized the familiar sound of American planes flying low overhead.

Late in the evening, as the sun was setting and the fighting continued, the sky lit up in a fiery cascade of flamingo colors. American tanks rolled up to the gates, and the ground began to shake and flares were fired into the air. Then, one tank burst through, followed by several others that drove into the courtyard.

They heard screams, "They're here! They're finally here!" A crowd of internees had gathered into the lobby, cheering around the soldiers that came out of the tanks. After what only seemed like a few minutes, a bomb blasted, and everyone took cover.

Suddenly, the Japanese started bombing outside of the university. When the tanks crashed through the front gate, the Japanese retreated to the education building with 200 internees who became their hostages. The American soldiers had to line up and return fire. After the Japanese decided things were not going well, the Americans began to negotiate with the Japanese soldiers. They negotiated their escape and the freedom of the Santo Tomas hostages.

I am not sure if the prisoners could sleep that night. At first, the negotiations failed and the Americans bombed part of the building. They finally decided that the remaining 47 Japanese soldiers would be escorted by our troops, with their arms in the air, and be released to a specific district that had been designated for the former captors.

The next morning, the prisoners rushed out to greet the American soldiers who had taken over control of the internment camp. Cheers ensued and candy bars where handed out to the kids. One can only imagine they were coming out of daze. Even though the United States Army came to free them, they still stayed in camp for the next several days while the fighting continued. One dear friend told me she felt safer and finally had hope because, for the first time the American soldiers were with them and protecting them.

345

Could there ever be a more trying testing ground for humankind than living in a foreign country in an internment camp? Human nature in a way must betray itself. Just prior to the outbreak of World War II, practically every American resident in Manila would have considered it incredible that little Japan could be a match for great, big America.

Following the broadcast of Pearl Harbor, the average American who had enjoyed the privileges of life in the Orient confidently made some such a remark: "It won't be long now until the little Japanese will hear from us." We all truly believed America would defeat Japan within a few weeks.

After three weary years of internment, their clothes in tatters, and after they had eaten their usual breakfast of grubby rice, they heard for the first time the welcome sound of the drone of American planes overhead. How hearts must have filled to overflowing tears, filling their eyes, albeit, tears of joy proclaiming they were free. After the shock of happy surprise, usually too deep for articulate expression, the internees would soon be going home to their families and friends. What a thrill to the ears of all who listened to the announcement made by General MacArthur himself, confirming that they indeed were saved.

At that time the war began, the Chinese and Americans did not know that day that the Battle of Manila would rage on for three more weeks, let alone three years. I was told they still had to remain in the Santo Tomas Internment Camp under MacArthur's orders, but there was to be no air strikes in order to protect the civilians in the ground war.

On February 6, MacArthur visited the camp to thousands of cheers and had planned to have a celebration parade, but shortly after he left, the Japanese shelling and fighting began in earnest for the next three days, and some of our liberated internees were killed and wounded. The Americans discovered that the Japanese

346

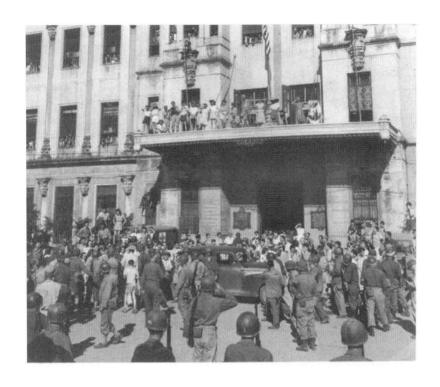

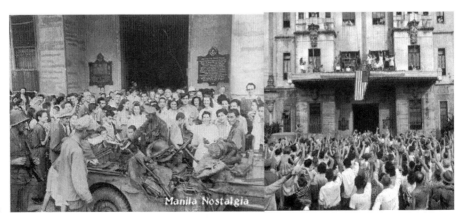

American soldiers arrive to liberate camps, February 1945

did not plan to give up Manila before destroying the whole city. This month-long battle was the second most destructive battle of all time.

While the Japanese fought the American soldiers in Manila, one of the greatest achievements was a carefully planned rescue operation that took place on February 23. Major Burgess and his troops rescued 2,000 Los Baños internees and lead them to San Antonio to their liberation.

By March 3, Manila, the once "Pearl of the Orient," was reduced to rubble after a month of the worst war combat ever known. General MacArthur had lost seventeen percent of his force of 35,000 men in addition to 3,000 Filipinos, and over 100 Filipino citizens lay dead in the rubble, known as the Manila massacre. Most were deliberately murdered by the Japanese troops that were on their last legs and desperate to take back the city.

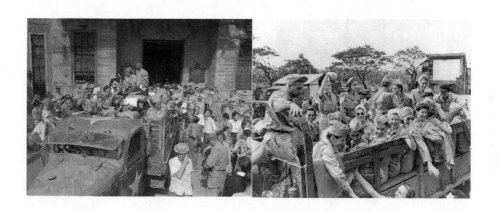

Freedom awaits the Santo Tomas internees, February 1945

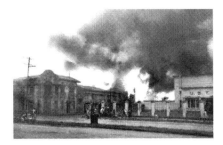

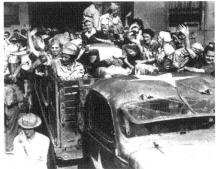

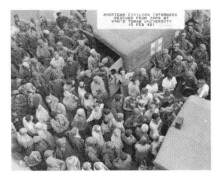

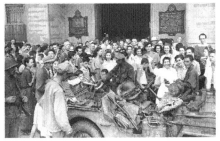

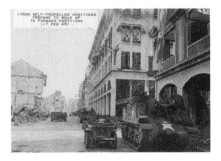

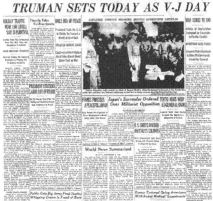

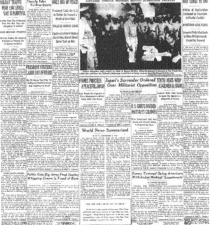

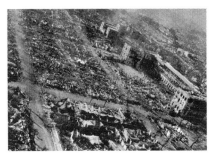

Chinese liberation of Santo Tomas internment camp and aftermath

I was relieved that the war was over, many of my fellow prisoners were saved and would soon be coming home to their loved ones, just as I had done thirteen months earlier. But even after the joyful liberation, there would be many months of sober recovery from such gruelling months of inhumane captivation and deprivation.

I did not realize then that the physical therapy work I did in the internment camps would be my swan song. While it was the most difficult and challenging time of my life, the one outstanding joy during that time was the enjoyment of helping others and providing service for no money and without price or equipment, performing without adequate food to keep our bodies' fires burning, and with little comfort, clothes, or hope.

I believed then, as I did until the end, that all physical therapists should always bring a sympathetic, understanding, and healthy judgment of how the mind, body, and spirit can heal their patients when under the care of a practitioner's good cheer, self-reliance, skill, and faith.

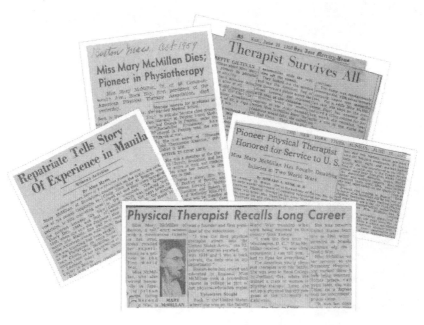

Newspaper articles about Mary McMillan as founder of Physical Therapy and survivor of the Japanese internment camps in World War II

350

PART FIVE
1944-1959

16

MARY MCMILLAN'S LEGACY

It took me over two years to recover after I returned from the camps and I decided to finally retire. At this time, I lived at 46 Commonwealth Avenue. It was nice to begin the last phase of my life when my health and my Scottish pride of spirit returned. I spent my time entertaining friends and colleagues and had weekly gatherings at my apartment in Boston, which was furnished with many of my Chinese treasures from the Orient. Guests would often bring me gifts and some of my Chinese visitors would bring me herbs and vitamins, as they were greatly concerned about my well-being.

As I reflected over the first 25 years of the American Physical Association, I felt we had gone through the birth pain of our profession and come to the place where our birth pains were now over. Even though my last therapy sessions were performed in a Japanese prison encampment, I had no regrets of letting go of the practice of physical therapy. I was now 65 years old and it was time to rest and heal my own body. My greatest hope was that I had been a guiding light on three continents—the United States, China, and the Philippines—during the war.

Even though I was sometimes suffering, I still believed I could do more to inspire and help the mission of physical therapy. I attended the meeting of physiotherapist at the army headquarters in Boston on Friday, January 28, 1944. I gave a talk on the need of their services. E.J. Brehaut, the Director of Officer Procurement, sent me a kind thank you note acknowledging my devotion to our profession and wishing me a speedy recovery from my illness with a long life of happiness.

I was awarded an honorary membership in the National Physical Therapy Association, the first honor to a physical therapist, and even though I was retired, my fingers kept busy, and on June 4, 1944, I wrote a paper on "New China in the Making" to the congregation of the Harvard Church. I still felt there was so much America could do to help China.

In September 1944, I attended the Congress of Physical Therapy in Chicago. I wrote another paper and delivered a talk on December 28, 1944 about "Traditional China is Changing" to the congregation of the Harvard Church.

On May 28, 1945, I received a letter from the National Foundation for Infantile Paralysis in New York from Catherine Worthingham, inviting me to attend scholarship ceremony. I decided to attend. I was pleased the APA changed its name to APTA on January 1, 1946, and created a House of Delegates. The House of Delegates was setup to continue the standards and legislative bylaws of the association in regards to physical therapy practices and the profession.

The passage of the Hospital Survey and Construction Act of 1946—the Hill-Burton Act—led to an increase in hospital-based practice for physical therapists. They wanted to be prepared and well staffed because in 1950, the Korean War again challenged United States Army physical therapists with the treatment of those with disabilities related to war wounds.

I gave another speech at the APTA conference in Boston in 1949, where I shared, "No, friends, it is not to me that credit or honor is due for the growth and development of the association. It is to the chapter presidents, past and present, the national officers, past and present, who meet at conventions and at other times from morning until late in the evening to help iron out our problems.

It is your directors, standing committees, advisory committees; it is to years of devoted service of executive director, secretary and staff, to those in the army who through the years have fought and won military status for army physical therapists. It is those, who for years, gave of their time and talents to make the *Physical Therapy Review* a success. It is to all these that I would like to honor. The National Association has given me so much and enriched my life exceedingly and made me very happy."

I was asked to speak at the opening session of the Massachusetts Chapter of Physical Therapy. I arrived in London, England, on March 10, 1950, on a Pan American flight. Air travel was new and I was happy to visit England one last time. While there, I learned that British Commonwealth countries began the practice of manipulative therapy for patients who had spine and joint issues. It was a new practice with combinations of exercise and manipulative therapy. It was at this time that physical therapy moved from being practiced just in hospitals to new rehab centers at schools, nursing facilities, and private doctor's offices.

When I returned from Europe on March 24, 1950, I moved to a new apartment located at 75 Chestnut Street in Boston, Massachusetts where my beloved sister Lizzie took great care of me. I was so happy to read, in a letter dated March 25, 1950 from Department of from Emma Vogel who was in the army office of the Surgeon General, letting me know that the legislation they had been working on since 1947 passed. The legislation finally acknowledged the benefits of therapists in the United States Army whereas before they were civilian status only.

During this time, our McMillan Scottish clan grew smaller when my brother, Edward Neil, died on April 3, 1951. I was 70 years old and in Los Angeles, California. My heart grieved for his loss, as it was another McMillan to pass into God's arms.

I was invited to the World Confederation for Physical Therapy at the Ingeniorhuset Restaurant in Copenhagen, Denmark, on

September 8, 1951, but did not feel well enough to attend. Eleven countries joined together: Australia, Canada, Denmark, Finland, Great Britain, New Zealand, Norway, South Africa, West Germany, Sweden, and the United States of America. Miss Mildred Elson represented the United States of America.

I was gratified to hear that in September 1953, the same year as the Queen's Coronation, 1,700 physical therapists came from 25 countries for the First International Congress of the World Confederation of Physical Therapy. I was unable to attend, but Mildred Olsen, and many dear colleagues I knew, attended and shared with delight how wonderful the event was.

Shortly thereafter, my half brother, Archibald Livingston, died on July 2, 1954 in Philadelphia, Pennsylvania, which hit our family hard in our hearts. Even though I had seen so much death in my life, when it happens close to home, it ages the soul.

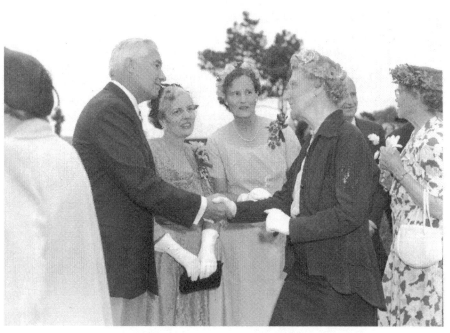

Mary McMillan lecturing after return from Japanese internment camps

On June 17, 1956, I rallied once again and attended the Second Congress of World Confederation. The wonderful event was held at the Statler Hotel in New York City and over 2,000 members attended the five-day conference. The ceremony opened at the Collegiate Church and I was the honored guest. I gave the opening ceremony speech and reflected over my many years of service in physical therapy.

I was pleased to receive a kind thank you letter on June 26, 1956 from my dear friend, Mildred Elson, who was the president of the organization, sharing what a wonderful life I had, loving and caring for my fellow man, and that I was a source of inspiration to all of the members of the World Confederation for Physical Therapy.

I still kept busy with writing and my correspondence. I attended a reception in February 1957 at Sargent College and gave a speech at the Pinning Ceremony. Afterwards, many of the students thanked me and said, "This is the inspiration we have been seeking," and "Now we understand the profession." Sadly, my dear brother, John William, died on December 7, 1957 in Pinehurst, North Carolina, and while I was not able to attend his funeral, I sent a nice condolence card to his family.

On October 24, 1959, it was my turn. I said goodbye to the world and passed peacefully away at home surrounded by my dear family and friends. My funeral had been carefully planned and was held at Harvard Church in Brookline on October 27. Before I passed, I shared that I had hoped and prayed that I would be remembered by all who knew me and that I was able to "carry our own weight, be of some service, and that I had learned to succor the unfortunate."

WORLD CONFEDERATION FOR PHYSICAL THERAPY
News

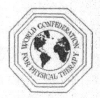

Second Congress

WORLD CONFEDERATION FOR PHYSICAL THERAPY

Date — June 17-23, 1956

Place — Hotel Statler, New York City

Program

The program has been developed around the theme "Health, A Strong Force for World Understanding — The Role of the Physical Therapist"

Sunday, June 17

A.M. Arrangements will be made for special religious services.

P.M. Registration — all tickets, final program, and other pertinent material will be distributed.
Welcoming Reception.

Monday, June 18

10:00 A.M. Opening Ceremony of the Congress.

11:30 A.M. Opening of exhibits.

2:00 P.M. Presentations of the status and needs of physical therapy by representatives of governments.

Tuesday through Friday, June 19-22

The scientific program will include presentations on

Anterior Poliomyelitis — The role of the physical therapist in the evaluation studies of the polio vaccine field trials.

Cerebral Palsy — Similarities and differences in methods of treatment.

Prosthetics — Recent research, prescription, fitting and training.

Bracing and Adaptive Devices for neuromuscular disorders.

Evaluation Procedures — Physical achievement, manual and electrical muscle tests, joint measurements.

Underwater Exercise — Physical principles and therapeutic use.

Posture Symposium.

Ultrasonics.

Physiological Basis for Heat.

Home and Convalescent Care Programs — including the severely disabled.

Antenatal and Postnatal Exercise.

The Physical Therapist — His education and responsibilities; his relationships to his fellow-workers and the community.

Seminar on Education.

A detailed program will be available later.

Film Theatre

Films of special interest to the members of the Congress will be selected.

Exhibits

Technical — Presentation of therapeutic exercise, electrical and hydrotherapy equipment; wheel chairs; crutches; braces; adaptive equipment; prosthetic appliances; textbooks, etc.

Scientific — Presentation of research and clinical studies related to the scientific program.

Social Program

A social event for each evening is being planned. This will include the official banquet, a boat trip around New York, receptions by the Canadian Physiotherapy Association, the American Physical Therapy Association, and the International Society for the Welfare of Cripples. Additional entertainment is being planned for the social associate members.

Study Tours and Visits

Arrangements will be made for visits to departments in New York City and environs, as well as in other cities in which colleagues may be visiting, immediately prior to or the week after Congress.

Two planned tours may be arranged of 5-7 days' duration — one to Boston and one to Washington. Stops would be made at intermediate points for sightseeing and hospital visits. Details will be available later.

Membership Categories

Full Members — Physical therapists, occupational therapists, medical social workers, physicians, vocational counsellors, nurses, administrators of hospitals and rehabilitation centers, board and staff members of organizations interested in the handicapped.

Student Members — Students in the approved schools of physical therapy in the member or-

388

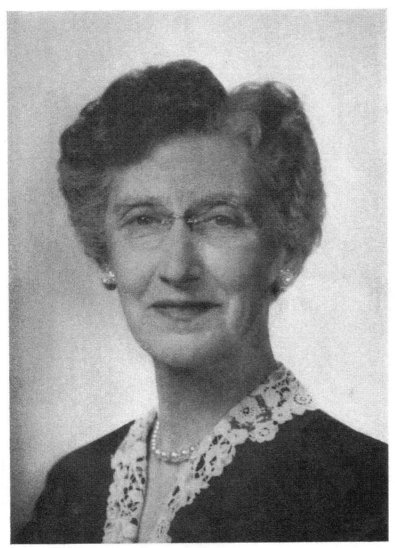

Mary McMillan
1880-1959

17

MARY MCMILLAN'S CONTRIBUTIONS TO PHYSICAL THERAPY

Mary McMillan died on October 29, 1959. She succumbed to long-term complications she contracted in the Santo Tomas and Chapei Internment Camps. She had metastatic melanoma due to the long hours of overexposure to the sun in the camps. She was loved and cherished by many and had taught many great life lessons. Mary shared her speech on the 25th Anniversary of the American Physical Therapy Association, entitled "Physical Therapy on Three Continents," and ended the lecture by sharing this story: "A girl about fourteen was referred to physical therapy from the camp clinic in the Santo Tomas Internment Camp with a diagnosis of painful tender feet. She was an adolescent girl whose whole appearance registered unhappiness. I tried to get her body in a little better alignment and she came in daily for treatments. One day she confided in me how she was feeling. I replied, 'I see by your actions and reactions that you are filled with bitterness and jealousy. You are a very pretty girl but you don't look pretty because your face reveals envy and bitterness.' I shared that psychiatrists had proven that these states of mind react unfavorably upon the physical body.

"Then I shared, 'There is not much use in working to improve your body until your mental attitude is changed toward your life.' I suggested that I needed someone to help me in my work and asked if she would help me. She said she would like to do so. Later, I was able to find work for her in the children's department of the hospital. She loved children and they adored her. Shortly thereafter, I left Santo Tomas for another internment camp.

"I wondered many times what had happened to the youngster. About eighteen months later, when I was aboard the ship, the MS Gripsholm, a very lovely girl came up to me and asked, with a sparkle in her eye, 'Have I improved any?' I replied, 'Natalie, I hardly recognized you.' Then she put her arms around me and hugged me, then said, 'I don't know what I would have done without you.'"

This personal story illustrates that Mary knew physical therapists do not have many chances to do the same thing, and not in the same way. She believed it is a requisite to have a sympathetic understanding of their patients. They must know when to give their patients the room to let off steam and to put in the right word. They should be healthy in body and mind, and cheerful, for these things were infectious. They ought to keep up with the latest in their profession so that when new things come along, they are aware of them so that they may be of the greatest service to their patients.

It is a necessity to believe in themselves, for without this, others cannot have faith in them. They are obliged to never show or allow their patients to lose hope—and she didn't mean false hope either. This was the essence of what Mary McMillan believed, illustrated, and taught. She believed the greatest gift you could give your patients was *real* hope because hope helps to chase fears away and is the greatest healer. When fears fade to perseverance, it gives a chance for nature's healing. Of course, it's not always easy. There will be hard knocks. It is the hard knocks that will bring out the best in us. It is how we deal with disappointment that will define our lives, our future, and our very legacy. She was often quoted as saying, "It's a hard job, but who wants a soft job anyway," and what harder job is there than giving people hope in the midst of their pain and suffering?

Mary McMillan's contributions to physical therapy endured for 50 years of her life and continue to this day. Many honors, writings, and articles memorialized her life and work after her death. Family, friends, and colleagues wrote hundreds of thank you cards, letters, and accounts of how much "Dear Mollie" meant to and inspired them to be happier, more self-realized, successful physical therapists, and compassionate human beings.

Examples of these letters were printed in the *Physical Therapy Review*, Volume 40, Number 2, and were published in June 1960, where twenty full pages honored Mary McMillan. These letters offer a sense of how admired, adored, appreciated, and valued she was by so many people.

***

"To talk with Mollie was, to me, a tonic. She was so proud of her association to the APTA. Never once did she ever show disappointment in our shortcomings. There was always encouragement, praise, and a thank you for our efforts even though they seemed to us to be feeble and ineffective. Another one of Mollie's strengths was her great sense of humor, which kept everything in balance. Life couldn't be grim when you talked with her. She would dispel one's concern by telling of her experiences with a twinkle in her eye and laughter in her voice."
—— *Mildred Wilson, Executive Director APTA, 1944-1956*

"She had great faith and held no resentment of bitter experience and met illness with great courage and reserve. This undoubtedly came from the great spiritual strength she gained from reserving a portion of each morning for reading the Bible, often excusing herself, Withdrawal apart to rest awhile…I shall never forget one time when I was feeling discouraged about making a change in my life. I had taken to heart Matthew 7:1: Judge not, that ye be not judged. Knowing there were always two sides to consider, Mollie instantly answered, 'Yes, my dear, but there is also verse seven: Ask, and it will be given unto you. And most assuredly a way will come.'" —— *Edith Munro, Sixth APTA President*

"*Mary was a remarkable woman who will go down in history as the 'Mother of Physical Therapy' and 'Founder of the American Physical Therapy Asso- ciation.'*" — Emma E. Vogel, United States Colonel and First Chief Women's Medical Specialist.

"*Mary was a marvelous combination of seriousness and fun. Very truly her life was given to the care and love of her fellow beings and the dear Lord must have had a very special niche for her life in His Kingdom.*" — Emily Griffin, World War II reconstruction aide and APTA Charter Member

"*My association with Mary was personal rather than professional. Two characteristics, which I especially associate with her, were her sincere interest in the welfare of others and her delightful sense of humor, which enabled others, as well as herself, to face difficult situations.*" — Ruth W. Dean, friend, Seattle, Washington

"*I wish every PT could appreciate how much her life has meant to the profession and to every one of us. We can be proud that our profession was organized by one with the high professional standards, which Mary McMillan possessed and practiced. It always distresses me to find a member who doesn't know of Mollie McMillan.*" — Gertrude Beard, Director of School of Physical Therapy, Fourth President of the APTA and Editor of the Physical Therapy Review "*Her joy and enthusiasm in her profession was as great in 1959 as it was when she began her studies in Liverpool in 1900. Her legacy to the members of the APTA is a living vital challenge.*

Would that we could all have, even in smaller amounts, her compassion and dedication, her wisdom and courtesy, her personal dignity and sense of humor, coupled with her sensitivity to people and situations, her belief in integrity for all people, and her vision to meet and solve perplexing problems and understanding."

— Mildred O. Olsen, First APTA Lecture

THE physical therapy REVIEW

37th Annual Conference
American Physical Therapy Association
Penn-Sheraton Hotel   Pittsburgh, Pennsylvania
June 26 — July 1, 1960

Volume 40, Number 2   **February 1960**

PUBLISHED MONTHLY BY
AMERICAN PHYSICAL THERAPY ASSOCIATION

18

THE MARY MCMILLAN APTA LECTURE AWARD AND SCHOLARSHIP

After Mary's death, it was revealed in her will that she left half of her substantial estate and fortune to the American Physical Therapy Association. A trust was left to assist and establish a scholarship in 1959, which would be worth over two million dollars today.

In 1963, the Mary McMillan Lecture Award was established to pay tribute to Mary McMillan, the pioneer of physical therapy, an esteemed teacher, and the founding member and first president of what is now known as the American Physical Therapy Association (APTA). The McMillan Lecture Award is the most distinguished honor an active member can receive.

The award is given to a physical therapist who has exhibited preeminent skills in administration, education, patient care, management, and research. The first award was given to Mildred O. Elson, a physical therapist who presented the first lecture, "The Legacy of Mary McMillan," on July 8, 1964.

The American Physical Therapy Association Mary McMillan Scholarship Award is bestowed to future physical therapists who are in their last year of their education and show excellent academic ability and professional viability that will be long-lasting. The first two Mary McMillan scholarship recipients were awarded in 1963 to Patricia A. McFarland and Elen McMahon.

A full list of the last 55 Mary McMillan Lecture Awards and over 350 Mary McMillan Scholarship Award winners are listed on the APTA website: www.apta.org. We would like to offer a special thanks and congratulations to the American Physical Therapy Association, which will turn 100 years old on January 15, 2021.

19
ACKNOWLEDGMENTS

O n behalf of Mary McMillan and her family, we would like to thank the following people for their help, encouragement, kindness, and support on Mary McMillan's official biography. Please learn more about Mary and share your stories at www.marymcmillan.com

On behalf of the author
Mary Farrell

I would like to thank Shirley Ross Davis for your support and believing in Mary McMillan's story. I am also grateful to Vesna Obradovic for your help in my preparation and research. Thank you to Kevin Farrell, Audrey Crevelt, Barbara Cray, Marian B Farrell (my mother, who always encouraged me to write), Elizabeth McMillan Buckley, my dear grandmother who saved all of Aunt Mollie's letters, diaries, documents, and stories for me to be able to share her sister's legacy (Mary McMillan) today. Bruce McMillan, Kathleen Thornton, Kelley Mcmanley, and Deborah Don who all helped to contribute their time and help with this project.

On behalf of the author
Marta M. Mobley

I would especially like to thank my loving and supportive husband, Nelson Miles Anderson, my sweet and encouraging children, Emma and Tessa Anderson. I'd like to offer my sincere gratitude to my life coach, Nancy Tylim, who has so gracefully guided me through so many of my greatest trials and triumphs. And a special note of gratitude to my dearest and beloved home-grown family; sister Christiana Musk and goddaughter Ryan Wyly, my Mamabear and mentor, Echo Bodine and adopted brother Tomas Kitchens and his Kitchen's family clan.

On behalf of the authors
Mary Farrell and Marta M. Mobley

A huge thank you to all those who helped make this book possible: Story Terrace (Ari Davine, Emily McCracken, Amanda Wilson, and Sam Brockschmidt); the American Physical Therapy Association, Sharon Dunn, Justin Moore, Gini Blodgett Birchett, and Megan H. Smith; as well as the United States Army, Reed College, Rockefeller Archive Center, the World Confederation for Physical Therapy, Freya Rodger; United Parish in Brookline (aka Harvard Church), Sarah Fitzpatrick; Congregational Church of Harvard, Susan Buck; Billo Billingsley tpcliverpool; David McMillan and George McMillan at www.clanmacmillan.org; Graeme Mackenzie; Jane Roone at the Huyton College Old Girls Guild and Liverpool College; Roger Hull-Liverpool Record Office; The Reed College Library-Laura Buchholz-Special Collections and Archives; Margret Parry, Library Assistant, Liverpool Record Office; Mrs. Maggie Willet, Business Manager, St. Michael in the Hamlet; Susan Bamber, Principal's PA-Liverpool College; Liberty Ellis Foundation; Flicker.com; Ancestry.com; Myheritage.com; Rootsweb.com; Findmypast.com; Familysearch.org; highlandroots. net; the City of Boston; all United States World War I and II prisoners of war;